An Atlas of
HEADACHE

THE ENCYCLOPEDIA OF VISUAL MEDICINE SERIES

An Atlas of
HEADACHE

Stephen D. Silberstein, MD
Jefferson Headache Center, Philadelphia, PA

Alan Stiles, DMD
Jefferson Headache Center, Philadelphia, PA

William B. Young, MD
Jefferson Headache Center, Philadelphia, PA

and

Todd D. Rozen, MD
Cleveland Clinic Foundation, Cleveland, OH

The Parthenon Publishing Group
International Publishers in Medicine, Science & Technology

A CRC PRESS COMPANY
BOCA RATON   LONDON   NEW YORK   WASHINGTON, D.C.

Library of Congress Cataloging-in-Publication Data
  Data available on request

Published in the USA by
The Parthenon Publishing Group
345 Park Avenue South, 10th Floor
New York, NY 10010, USA

Published in the UK and Europe by
The Parthenon Publishing Group
23–25 Blades Court
Deodar Road
London SW15 2NU, UK

British Library Cataloguing-in-Publication Data
An atlas of headache. - (The encyclopedia of visual
medicine series)
  1. Headache
  I. Silberstein, Stephen D.
  616.8′491

ISBN 185070547X

Copyright © 2002 The Parthenon Publishing Group

Typeset by Siva Math Setters, Chennai, India
Printed and bound by T.G. Hostench S.A., Spain

Contents

List of contributors

Stephen D. Silberstein, MD
Jefferson Headache Center
111 S. 11th Street
Suite 8130 Gibbon Bldg
Philadelphia, PA 19107

William B. Young, MD
Jefferson Headache Center
111 S. 11th Street
Suite 8130 Gibbon Bldg
Philadelphia, PA 19107

Mario F. P. Peres, MD
Sao Paulo Headache Center
R. Maestro Cardim, 887
01323–001
Sao Paulo
Brazil

Alan Stiles, DMD
Jefferson Headache Center
111 S. 11th Street
Suite 8130 Gibbon Bldg
Philadelphia, PA 19107

Todd D. Rozen, MD
Cleveland Clinic Foundation
Department of Neurology T33
9500 Euclid Avenue
Cleveland, OH 44195

Charles Siow, MD
Jefferson Headache Center
111 S. 11th Street
Suite 8130 Gibbon Bldg
Philadelphia, PA 19107

Acknowledgements

Nitamar Abdala, MD
Federal University of Sao Paulo
Rua Napoleao de Barros, 800
Vila Clementino
Sao Paulo, SP, CEP 04024–002
Brazil

David J. Capobianco, MD
Mayo Clinic, Jacksonville
4500 San Pablo Road
Jacksonville, FL 32224

Gary Carpenter, MD
Jefferson Medical College
1025 Walnut Street
Philadelphia, PA 19107

Henrique Carrete Jr, MD
Department of Radiology
Universidade Federal de São Paulo
São Paulo
Brazil

John Edmeads, MD
Sunnybrook Medical Center
University of Toronto
2075 Bayview Avenue
Toronto, Ontario M4N 3M5
Canada

Peter J. Goadsby, MD
Institute of Neurology
National Hospital for Neurology &
    Neurosurgery
Queen Square
London WC1N 3BG
United Kingdom

Richard Hargreaves, PhD
Pharmacology and Imaging
Merck Research Laboratories
Merck & Co, Inc
WP 42–300
770 Sumneytown Pike
P.O. Box 4
West Point, PA 19486

Bernadette Jaeger, DDS
Section of Oral Medicine and Orofacial Pain
School of Dentistry
University of California, Los Angeles
Los Angeles, CA 90064–1782

Marco A. Lana-Peixoto, MD
Federal University of Minas Gerais
    Medical School
Rua Psdre Rolim 769–13 Andar
Belo Horizonte - MG 30130–090
Brazil

Richard B. Lipton, MD
Innovative Medical Research
1200 High Ridge Road
Stamford, CT 06905

Suzana M.F. Malheiros, MD
Department of Neurology
Universidade Federal de São Paulo
São Paulo
Brazil

Pericles de Andrade Maranhao-Filho,
   MD, MSc, PhD
Federal University of Rio de Janeiro
Clementino Fraga Filho Hospital
National Institute of Cancer
Rio de Janeiro
Brazil

Andrew A. Parsons, PhD
Head Migraine & Stroke Research
GlaxoSmithKline
Neurology Centre of Excellence
   for Drug Discovery
New Frontiers Science Park
Harlow, Essex
United Kingdom

Julio Pascual, MD
University Hospital 'Marqués de Valdecilla'
39008 Santander
Spain

Luiz Paulo de Queiroz, MD, MSc
Clinica do Cerebro
Rua Presidente Coutinho, 464
88015–231 Florianopolis, SC
Brazil

Margarita Sanchez del Rio, MD
Neurology Department
Fundacion Hospital Alcorcon
Juan Carlos I University
Alcorcon, Madrid,
Spain

Germany Goncalves Veloso, MD
Department of Neurology
Federal University of Sao Paulo
Sao Paulo
Brazil

Paul Winner, DO, FAAN
Palm Beach Headache Center
Nova Southeastern University
5205 Greenwood Avenue
West Palm Beach, FL 33407

Vera Lucia Faria Xavier, MD
Headache Center
Santo Amaro University
Sao Paulo
Brazil

Foreword

In medieval maps, the periphery of the world was shrouded in mystery with vivid images of hypothetical dragons lurking at the edges. One might suspect that an 'Atlas of Headache' would be rife with such dragons as not all of the headache world has been completely charted. How does one see a headache? How does one map a headache?

The present authors are to be commended for presenting an 'Illustrated Headache News' for our information and enjoyment. The common headache entities of migraine, cluster and tension-type headaches as well as the more sinister structural causes of headache are outlined in the text to provide a framework on which to hang the illustrations – some scientific, some historical and some artistic. This display makes for a relaxed approach to a complex subject like ambling through an art gallery to view an exhibition that conveys a message. It is a pathway well worth taking for pleasure as well as enlightenment.

James W. Lance
Emeritus Professor of Neurology
University of New South Wales
Sydney, Australia
President of the International
Headache Society, 1987–9

Preface

Physicians need to learn to diagnose and manage headaches. Despite this need, it is rare for medical students to have more than one lecture on headache management during their education, and residents in training, even in neurology, rarely get any more formal training. Educating caregivers to recognize head pain complaints will provide better care for patients.

Our Atlas approaches the problem of headache from a visual perspective; it visualizes the subjective complaint of headache and makes it easier to understand. For some, this type of visual learning may be the best approach; for others, it will reinforce other learning strategies. Anything that leads to a better understanding of headaches will lead to better diagnosis and management.

There are many causes of headache. Some are secondary to other conditions; others are disorders in themselves. Diagnosis and treatment is often a challenge. We include the history of headache, its epidemiology, diagnosis and treatment. We address migraine, tension-type and cluster headache, in addition to the rare or more unusual primary and secondary headache disorders. We have tried to include classic images from other texts, as well as new images that illustrate the disorders and reflect the most current thinking. This compilation of images has been contributed by physicians from all over the world. Our goal in presenting an overview of the numerous disorders that cause head pain is to provide a better understanding for those treating these disorders and, ultimately, better care for headache sufferers.

Stephen D. Silberstein, Alan Stiles,
William B. Young and Todd D. Rozen
April 2002

Section I A Review of Headache

CHAPTER 1

Historical aspects of headache

HEADACHE IN THE ANCIENT WORLD

Headache has troubled mankind from the dawn of civilization. Signs of trepanation, a procedure wherein the skull was perforated with an instrument, are evident on neolithic human skulls dating from 7000–3000 BC[1] (Figures 1.1 and 1.2). Originally, it was thought that the procedure had been performed to release demons and evil spirits, but recent evidence suggests that it was carried out for medical reasons[2]. Trepanation continues to be practiced today, without anesthesia, by some African tribes. It is primarily performed for relief of headache or removal of a fracture line after head injury[3].

Headache prescriptions written on papyrus (Figure 1.3) were already known in ancient Egypt. The Ebers Papyrus, dated circa 1200 BC and said to be based on medical documents from 2500 BC, describes migraine, neuralgia and shooting head pains[4]. It was practice at the time to firmly bind a clay crocodile holding grain in its mouth to the patient's head using a strip of linen that bore the names of the gods[5,6] (Figure 1.4). This technique may have produced headache relief by compressing and cooling the scalp[5].

Hippocrates (470–410 BC, Figure 1.5) described a shining light, usually in the right eye, followed by violent pain that began in the temples and eventually reached the entire head and neck area[5]. He believed that headache could be triggered by exercise or intercourse[6], that migraine resulted from vapors rising from the stomach to the head

and that vomiting could partially relieve the pain of headache[5,6]. Celsus (215–300 AD) believed 'drinking wine, or crudity [dyspepsia] or cold, or heat of a fire or the sun' could trigger migraine. Because of his classic descriptions, Aretaeus of Cappodocia (second century AD) is credited with discovering migraine headache. The term 'migraine' itself is derived from the Greek word 'hemicrania', introduced by Galen in approximately 200 AD. He mistakenly believed it was caused by the ascent of vapors, either excessive, too hot or too cold. Clearly, migraine was well known in the ancient world[4].

HEADACHE OVER THE CENTURIES

In the twelfth century, Abbess Hildegarde of Bingen described her visions (Figure 1.6), later attributed to her migraine aura, in terms that are both mystical and apocalyptic[7]:

> 'I saw a great star, most splendid and beautiful, and with it an exceeding multitude of falling sparks with which the star followed southward … and suddenly they were all annihilated, being turned into black coals … and cast into the abyss so that I could see them no more'.

In 1683 Thomas Willis (Figures 1.7 and 1.8) brilliantly described a woman with severe, periodic, migrainous headache preceded by a prodrome and associated with vomiting[4]:

'... beautiful and young woman, imbued with a slender habit of body, and an hot blood, was wont to be afflicted with frequent and wandering fits of headache ... On the day before the coming of the spontaneous fit of this disease, growing very hungry in the evening, she eat a most plentiful supper, with an hungry, I may say a greedy appetite; presaging by this sign, that the pain of the head would most certainly follow the next morning; and the event never failed this augury .∴. she was troubled also with vomiting'.

Migraine was distinguished from common headache by Tissot in 1783[8], who ascribed it to a supraorbital neuralgia '... provoked by reflexes from the stomach, gallbladder or uterus'. Over the next century, DuBois Reymond, Mollendorf and, later, Eulenburg proposed different vascular theories for migraine. In the late eighteenth century, Erasmus Darwin (Figure 1.9), grandfather of Charles Darwin, suggested treating headache by centrifugation. He believed headaches were caused by vasodilation, and suggested placing the patient in a centrifuge to force the blood from the head to the feet[5,6]. Fothergill in 1778 introduced the term 'fortification spectra' to describe the typical visual aura or disturbance of migraine. Fothergill used the term 'fortification'[6] because the visual aura resembled a fortified town surrounded with bastions[9,10].

In 1873, Liveing (Figure 1.10) wrote the first monograph on migraine, entitled *On Megrim, Sick-headache, and Some Allied Disorders: A Contribution to the Pathology of Nerve-storms*, and originated the neural theory of migraine. He ascribed the problem to '... disturbances of the autonomic nervous system', which he called 'nerve storms'[9]. William Gowers, in 1888, published an influential neurology textbook, *A Manual of Disease of the Nervous System*[10]. Gowers emphasized the importance of a healthy lifestyle and advocated using a solution of nitroglycerin (1% in alcohol), combined with other agents, to treat headaches. The remedy later became known as the 'Gowers mixture'. Gowers was also famous for recommending Indian hemp (marijuana) for headache relief[5,6].

Lewis Carroll described migrainous phenomena in *Alice in Wonderland* and *Through the Looking Glass*, depicting instances of central scotoma, tunnel vision, phonophobia, vertigo, distortions in body image, dementia and visual hallucinations (Figures 1.11 and 1.12).

Greek and Roman ancient writings include references to 'blighted grains' and 'blackened bread', and to the use of concoctions of powdered barley flower to hasten childbirth. During the Middle Ages, written accounts of ergot poisoning first appeared. Epidemics were described in which the characteristic symptom was gangrene of the feet, legs, hands and arms, often associated with burning sensations in the extremities. The disease was known as 'Ignis Sacer' or 'Holy Fire' and, later, as 'St. Anthony's Fire', in honor of the saint at whose shrine relief was obtained. This relief probably resulted from the use of a diet free of contaminated grain during the pilgrimage to the shrine (Figure 1.13)[11]. The term 'ergot' is derived from the French word 'argot' meaning 'rooster's spur'. It describes the small, banana-shaped sclerotium of the fungus. Louis René Tulasne of Paris in 1853 established that ergot was not a hypertrophied rye seed, but a fungus having three stages in one life cycle, and he named it *Claviceps purpurea* (Figure 1.14). Once infected by the fungus, the rye seed was transformed into a spur-shaped mass of fungal pseudotissue, purple-brown in colour: the resting stage of the fungus, known as the 'sclerotium' (derived from the Greek 'skleros' meaning 'hard')[11]. In 1831, Heinrich Wiggers (Figure 1.15), a pharmacist of Göttingen, Germany tested ergot extracts in animals. Among his models was the 'rooster comb test': a rooster, when fed ergotin, became ataxic and nauseous, acquired a blanched comb and suffered from severe convulsions, dying days later. The 'rooster comb test' continued to be used into the following century by investigators studying the physiologic properties of ergot[11]. Later Woakes, in 1868, reported the use of ergot of rye in the treatment of neuralgia[12]. The earliest reports in the medical literature on the use of ergot in the treatment of migraine were those of Eulenberg in Germany in 1883, Thomson in the United States in 1894 and Campbell in England in 1894. Stevens' *Modern Materia Medica* mentioned the use of ergot for the treatment of migraine in 1907[13].

The first pure ergot alkaloid, ergotamine, was isolated by Stoll (Figure 1.16) in 1918 and used primarily in obstetrics and gynecology until 1925, when Rothlin successfully treated a case of severe and intractable migraine with a subcutaneous injection of ergotamine tartrate. This indication was pursued vigorously by various researchers over the following decades and was reinforced by the belief in a vascular origin of migraine and the concept that ergotamine tartrate acted as a vasoconstrictor. In 1938, John Graham and Harold Wolff[14] demonstrated that ergotamine worked by constricting blood vessels and used this as proof of the vascular theory of migraine (Figures 1.17 and 1.18).

For further milestones in the history of headache, see Figures 1.19–1.30.

MODERN HEADACHE TREATMENTS

The modern approach to treating migraine began with the development of sumatriptan by Pat Humphrey and his colleagues[15]. Based on the concept that serotonin can relieve headache, they designed a chemical entity that was similar to serotonin, although more stable and with fewer side-effects. This development led to the modern clinical trials for acute migraine treatment and to the elucidation of the mechanism of action of what are now called the triptans.

We are at the threshold of an explosion in the understanding, diagnosis and treatment of migraine and other headaches. Many new triptans have been developed and many more will soon be, or are already, available, including zolmitriptan, naratriptan, eletriptan, frovatriptan, rizatriptan and almotriptan. Modern preventive treatment began with the belief that migraine was due to excess serotonin. Sicuteri[16] helped develop methysergide, a serotonin antagonist, for the prophylactic treatment of migraine and cluster headache. After a long hiatus, new drugs are being tested and developed for the preventive treatment of migraine. The anti-epileptic drugs have been investigated and some have already been proven to be effective for migraine. Concomitant with the development of new treatments is the development of the basic sciences of headache and the renewed dedication of clinicians to headache treatment and teaching.

REFERENCES

1. Lyons A, Petrucelli RJ. *Medicine: An Illustrated History*. New York: Harry N. Abrams, Inc, 1978:113–5
2. Venzmer G. *Five Thousand Years of Medicine*. New York: Taplinger Publishing Co, 1972:19
3. Rawlings CE, Rossitch E. The history of trepanation in Africa with a discussion of its current status and continuing practice. *Surg Neurol* 1994;41:507–13
4. Critchley M. Migraine: From Cappadocia to Queen Square. In: Smith R, ed. *Background to Migraine*, Volume 1. London: Heinemann, 1967
5. Edmeads J. The treatment of headache: a historical perspective. In: Gallagher RM, ed. *Therapy for Headache*. New York: Marcel Dekker Inc, 1990:1–8
6. Lance JW. *Mechanisms and Management of Headache*, 4th edn. London: Butterworth Scientific, 1982:1–6
7. Singer C. The visions of Hildegarde of Bingen. In: Anonymous. *From Magic to Science*. New York: Dover, 1958
8. Sacks O. *Migraine: Understanding a Common Disorder*. Berkeley: University of California Press, 1985:158–9
9. Patterson SM, Silberstein SD. Sometimes Jello helps: perceptions of headache etiology, triggers and treatment in literature. *Headache* 1993;33:76–81
10. Raskin NH. Migraine: clinical aspects. In: *Headache*, 2nd edn. New York: Churchill-Livingstone, 1988: 35–98
11. Bové FJ. *The Story of Ergot*. New York: Karger, 1970
12. Woakes E. On ergot of rye in the treatment of neuralgia. *Br Med J* 1868;2:360–1
13. Silberstein SD. The pharmacology of ergotamine and dihydroergotamine. *Headache* 1997;37:S15–S25
14. Graham JR, Wolff HG. Mechanisms of migraine headache and action of ergotamine tartrate. *Arch Neurol Psychiatry* 1938;39:737–63
15. Humphrey PP, Feniuk W, Marriott AS, *et al.* Preclinical studies on the anti-migraine drug, sumatriptan. *Eur Neurol* 1991;31:282–90
16. Sicuteri F. Prophylactic and therapeutic properties of 1-methylsergic acid butanole in migraine. *Int Arch Allergy* 1959;15:300–7

CHAPTER 2

Headache classification

Headache, like any other disease entity, requires a classification system. Diagnosis of the various headache disorders will be more accurate and universal when it has as its basis a consistent classification system and a set of scientifically derived diagnostic criteria. The ideal classification table should be sensitive, specific, exhaustive, generalizable, reliable and valid. Sensitivity occurs when patients with a particular form of headache are all diagnosed as such; specificity is when patients who do not have a particular disorder are invariably excluded. A classification table is exhaustive when its usage enables all headaches to be classified. It is generalizable when it can be used in diverse settings by both headache specialist and non-specialist alike. Reliability occurs when the system has high inter-obsever repeatability with low variability. High correlation of diagnosis with the underlying biological disorder underlines validity.

The precusor to the modern classification was created in the early 1960s by an ad hoc committee of the United States National Institutes of Health[1]. The classification table it devised was an advancement to the scientific study of headache but at the same time was criticized by many as being too vague in its definitions. In 1985, the International Headache Society (IHS) formed a headache classification committee that published, in 1988, a classification system that has become the standard for headache diagnosis, particularly for clinical research[2]. The IHS criteria, as it soon became known, have since received broad international support and have been endorsed by the World Health Organization (WHO) and its principles incorporated into the International Classification of Diseases (ICD-10)[3]. In it, headaches are subtyped using the principles of classification developed by the American Psychiatric Association and assigned into 12 major categories (Figure 2.1). These can be divided into two broad groups, the primary headache disorders (categories 1–4) and the secondary headache disorders (categories 5–12). The primary headache disorders are classified based on symptom profiles, while the secondary headache disorders are classified based on their causes, e.g. metabolic, structural or vascular causes. The IHS system is currently undergoing revision.

REFERENCES

1. Ad Hoc Committee on Classification of Headache. Classification of headache. *JAMA* 1962;179:717–8
2. Headache Classification Committee of the International Headache Society. Classification and diagnostic criteria for headache disorders, cranial neuralgias and facial pain. *Cephalalgia* 1988;8 (Suppl 7):1–96
3. World Health Organisation. *The International Statistical Classification of Diseases and Related Health Problems*; 10th rev. Geneva: World Health Organisation, 1992–1994

CHAPTER 3

Epidemiology of migraine

INTRODUCTION

Headaches are one of the most common complaints encountered by the practicing physician. Despite the amount of suffering and disability they cause, headaches are still underdiagnosed and under-treated.

Epidemiology has important implications for the diagnosis and treatment of headache disorders. Examination of sociodemographic, distribution, impact, familial and environmental risk factors may provide clues to preventive strategies and disease mechanisms. In this chapter, epidemiologic terms, prevalence rates, impact, costs and comorbitity of migraine are reviewed.

DEFINITIONS OF EPIDEMIOLOGIC TERMS

For clinical practice and epidemiologic research, it is important to have precise definitions to enable reliable and valid diagnosis (Figure 3.1). Since there is no true diagnostic gold standard for the primary headache disorders, it is difficult to study validity and to define diagnostic boundaries for symptom-based conditions.

Epidemiologic studies often focus on prevalence or incidence. Prevalence is the proportion of a given population that has a disorder over a defined period of time. Lifetime prevalence is the proportion of individuals who have ever had the condition, and one-year prevalence is the proportion of individuals who have had at least one attack within one year. Incidence is the onset of new cases of a disease in a defined population over a given period of time.

EPIDEMIOLOGY OF PRIMARY AND SECONDARY HEADACHES

Using the IHS criteria, Rasmussen et al.[1] examined the population distribution of all headache disorders via in-person clinical assessment in a large, representative community sample in the greater Copenhagen area. The lifetime prevalence of tension-type headache was 78% and that of migraine 16%. The most common secondary cause was fasting, which was the case in 19% of patients, followed by nose/sinus disease in 15% of patients and head trauma in 4%. Non-vascular intracranial disease, including brain tumor, accounted for 0.5%. Rasmussen and Olesen[2] studied the epidemiology of other headache disorders. Lifetime prevalence of idiopathic stabbing headache was 2%, external compression headache was 4% and cold stimulus headache was 15%. Benign cough headache, benign exertional headache and headache associated with sexual activity were each 1%. Lifetime prevalence of hangover headache was 72%, of fever headache 63% and of headache associated with disorders of the nose or sinuses 15%. Headaches associated with severe structural lesions were rare. Most headaches showed a significant female predominance. Symptomatic headaches were more prevalent among migraineurs. In subjects with tension-type headache, only hangover headache was over-represented. There was no association between the headache disorders and abnormal routine blood chemistries or arterial hypertension. In women with migraine, however, diastolic blood pressure was significantly higher than in women without migraine.

MIGRAINE

Migraine is a very common condition worldwide. Estimates of its prevalence have varied widely, ranging from 3% to about 22% (Figure 3.2). The differences can be accounted for by the differing definitions and methodologies employed. A reasonable estimate of one-year prevalence of migraine in adults is 10 to 12% (6% in men and 15–18% in women). In a Danish epidemiologic study[3], lifetime prevalence of migraine was 16% (8% in men and 25% in women) and one-year prevalence was 10% (6% in men and 15% in women). Prevalence of migraine without aura was 6% and that of migraine with aura was 4%.

In the US population, the one-year prevalence of migraine was 12% (6% in men and 18% in women)[4]. The same rates were found in France[5]. Migraine has been estimated to affect 1.5% of people in Hong Kong, 2.6% in Saudi Arabia, and 3% in Ethiopia. In Japan and Malaysia, prevalence rates were similar to those found in Western countries (8.4 and 9.0%, respectively; Figure 3.3). A recent epidemiologic study in South America[6] showed one-year prevalence of migraine in women (men) of 17% (8) in Brazil, 6% (4) in Argentina, 14% (5) in Colombia, 12% (4) in Mexico and 12% (5) in Venezuela.

Migraine prevalence is age- and gender-dependent. Before puberty, migraine is slightly more common in boys, with the highest incidence between 6–10 years of age. In women, the incidence is highest between 14–19 years of age. In general, women are more commonly affected than men (Figure 3.4), with a lifetime prevalence of 12–17% and 4–6%, respectively. In the American Migraine Study, the one-year prevalence of migraine increased with age among women and men, reaching the maximum at ages 35–45 and declining thereafter (Figures 3.5 and 3.6). Migraine

prevalence is inversely proportional to income, with the low income groups having the highest prevalence (Figure 3.7). Ethnicity and geographic region also influence migraine prevalence[4]. It is highest in North America and Western Europe, and more prevalent among Caucasians than African- or Asian-Americans. Migraine is influenced by environmental and genetic factors. Migraine with aura has a stronger genetic influence than migraine without aura and is influenced more by environmental factors. Behavioral, emotional and climatologic changes may trigger migraine, modify the vulnerability to migraine or impact on its prevalence.

Evidence suggests that the incidence of migraine may be increasing. Stang et al.[7], in a population-based survey of migraine conducted from 1979–1981 in Olmsted County, found that there was a striking increase in the age-adjusted incidence of migraine in those under 45 years of age. Migraine incidence increased by 34% for women and by 100% for men. In this study, the overall age-adjusted incidence was 137 per 100 000 individuals per year for men and 294 per 100 000 individuals per year for women.

In contrast, the American Migraine Study II, a follow-up to the original American Migraine Study, showed that the prevalence of migraine in the United States is 18.2% for women and 6.5% for men. This is essentially unchanged from the original study (prevalence 17.6% and 5.7%, respectively). The distribution of disease by sociodemographic factors has remained stable over the last decade, and migraine continues to be more prevalent in Caucasians than in other ethnic groups and in the lower income groups.

Impact and costs

Migraine is a public health problem of enormous scope that has an impact on both the individual sufferer and on society. Migraine is a lifelong, common disorder that affects people during their most productive years. The individual burden accounts for the impact of attacks on quality of life, and reduction of family, social and recreational activities. The societal burden refers to direct costs, primarily the cost of medical care, and indirect costs, which are due to the impact on work (absenteeism and reduced effectiveness; Figure 3.8). The American Migraine Study estimates that 23 million US residents have severe migraine headaches. Twenty-five percent of women experience four or more severe attacks a month; 35% experience one to three severe attacks a month; and 40% experience one, or less than one, severe attack a month. Similar frequency patterns were observed for men[4].

In the American Migraine Study, more than 85% of women and more than 82% of men with severe migraine had some headache-related disability. About one-third were severely disabled or needed bed rest (Figure 3.9). As headache pain intensity increases, more migraineurs report disability (Figure 3.10). It is estimated that the typical male migraineur has 3.8 and the typical woman sufferer 5.6 days of bed rest each year, resulting in a total of 112 million bedridden days per year in the US[8]. In addition to the attack-related disability, many migraineurs live in fear, knowing that at any time an attack could disrupt their ability to work, care for their families or meet social obligations. In a prospective diary study, 17% of social and family activities had to be cancelled because of headaches[9].

Migraine has an enormous impact on society. In the US, annual lost productivity due to migraine costs 13 billion dollars[3], while direct costs are estimated to be 2.5 billion dollars per year. Migraine's impact on health care utilization is marked as well. The National Ambulatory Medical Care Survey, conducted from 1976–1977, found that 4% of all visits to physicians' offices (over 10 million visits a year) were for headache. Migraine also results in major utilization of emergency rooms and urgent care centers[10].

Comorbidity

Comorbidity refers to the coexistence of one disorder with another that occurs more commonly than by chance. Stroke, epilepsy, depression, mania, anxiety and panic disorders are comorbid with migraine. Comorbidity has implications for headache diagnosis. Migraine has substantial overlap of symptoms with its comorbid conditions.

Both epilepsy and migraine can cause headache and transient alterations of consciousness. Stroke and migraine can both cause transient neurologic signs and headaches. Prodromal migraine symptoms, such as fatigue and irritability, may be part of comorbid depression. Migraine is also a risk factor for a number of comorbid disorders. Comorbidity has important therapeutic implications. Comorbid conditions may impose therapeutic limitations, but therapeutic opportunities may arise as well. For example, anti-depressants would be the first option when migraine and depression are concomitant.

In addition to the diagnostic and therapeutic implications, the presence of comorbidity may provide clues to the pathophysiology of migraine. When two conditions occur in the same person, the apparent associations may arise by coincidence, one condition may cause the other or shared environmental or genetic risk factors might account for the co-occurrence of two disorders. For example, head injury is a risk factor for both migraine and epilepsy and may account for part of the relationship between the disorders. Shared genetic risk factors may also account for the association between comorbid disorders. Finally, independent genetic or environmental risk factors may produce a brain state that gives rise to both migraine and a comorbid condition.

Migraine and stroke

Both migraine and stroke are neurologic disorders that are associated with focal, neurologic signs, alterations in blood flow or headache. The relationship between stroke and migraine could be better understood by the following proposed classification system: (i) coexisting stroke and migraine; (ii) stroke with clinical features of migraine (symptomatic migraine, migraine mimic); (iii) migraine-induced stroke (with and without risk factors); (iv) uncertain[11]. The proportion of strokes attributed to migraine varies from 1–17% in clinical series. Migraine is a risk factor for stroke. The risk of stroke among women under 45 years of age with migraine was three-fold higher than that of controls, and six-fold higher than that of controls for women suffering migraine with aura. Young women with migraine who smoked increased their stroke risk to approximately ten-fold that of controls, and to 14-fold that of controls if they were on oral contraceptives[12].

Migraine and epilepsy

The prevalence of epilepsy in migraine patients is 5.9%, greatly exceeding the population prevalence of 0.5%. There is a two-fold increase in migraine among both epileptic probands and their relatives[13] (Figure 3.11). The comorbidity of migraine and epilepsy can be explained by a state of neuronal excitability that increases the risk of both disorders. Treatment strategies for patients with comorbid migraine and epilepsy may have limitations, such as drugs that lower seizure threshold (tricyclic antidepressants, neuroleptics), but anticonvulsants (topiramate, divalproex) are drugs of choice for this association.

Migraine and psychiatric disorders

Several population-based studies have examined the comorbidity of migraine, major depression, panic disorder and other psychiatric disorders. Stewart et al.[14] found that 15% of women and 12.8% of men with headache between the ages of 24–29 years had panic disorder. Migraine headache was higher in individuals with a history of panic disorder. The relative risk was 7.0 for men and 3.7 in women.

Merikangas et al.[15] found that anxiety and affective disorders were more common in migraineurs. The odds ratio was 2.2 for depression, 2.9 for bipolar spectrum disorders, 2.7 for generalized anxiety disorder, 3.3 for panic disorder, 2.4 for simple phobia and 3.4 for social phobia. Major depression and anxiety disorders were commonly found together. In individuals with all three disorders, the onset of anxiety generally precedes the onset of migraine, whereas the onset of major depression usually follows the onset of migraine.

Breslau et al.[16] found that lifetime rates of affective and anxiety disorders were elevated in migraineurs. After adjusting for sex, the odds ratios were 4.5 for major depression, 6.0 for manic episode, 3.2 for any anxiety disorder and 6.6 for panic disorder. Migraine with aura was more strongly associated with the various psychiatric disorders than was migraine without aura.

Personality disorders have been linked to migraine. Brandt et al.[17] used the Eysenck Personality Questionnaire (EPQ) in the Washington County Migraine Prevalence Study sample. The EPQ is a well-standardized measure that includes four scales: psychoticism (P), extroversion (E), neuroticism (N) and lie (L). Migraineurs had higher scores than controls on the EPQ N scale, indicating that they were more tense, anxious and depressed than the control group. Women with migraine scored significantly higher than controls on the P scale, indicating that they were more hostile, less interpersonally sensitive and out of step with their peers.

Chronic daily headache, particularly chronic migraine, is highly comorbid with depression, anxiety and insomnia[18]. Fibromyalgia is present in 35% of chronic migraine patients, and it is associated with depression and insomnia[19].

REFERENCES

1. Rasmussen BK, Jensen R, Schroll M, Olesen J. Epidemiology of headache in a general population – a prevalence study. *J Clin Epidemiol* 1991;44:1147–57

2. Rasmussen BK, Olesen J. Symptomatic and non-symptomatic headaches in a general population. *Neurology* 1992;42:1225–31

3. Russell MB, Rasmussen BK, Thorvaldsen P, Olesen J. Prevalence and sex-ratio of the subtypes of migraine. *Int J Epidemiol* 1995;24:612–8

4. Stewart WF, Lipton RB, Celentano DD, Reed ML. Prevalence of migraine headache in the United States. *JAMA* 1992;267:64–9

5. Henry P, Michel P, Brochet B, *et al.* A nationwide survey of migraine in France: prevalence and clinical features in adults. GRIM. *Cephalalgia* 1992;12:229–37

6. Morillo LE, Sanin LC, Takeuchi Y, *et al.* Headache in Latin America: A multination population-based survey. *Neurology* 2001;56:A544 (abstract)

7. Stang PE, Yanagihara PA, Swanson JW, *et al.* Incidence of migraine headache: a population-based study in Olmsted County, Minnesota. *Neurology* 1992; 42:1657–62

8. Hu XH, Markson LE, Lipton RB, *et al*. Burden of migraine in the United States: disability and economic costs. *Arch Intern Med* 1999;159:813–8

9. Edmeads J, Findlay H, Tugwell P, *et al*. Impact of migraine and tension-type headache on life-style, consulting behavior, and medication use: a Canadian population survey. *Can J Neurol Sci* 1993;20:131–7

10. Celentano DD, Stewart WF, Lipton RB, Reed ML. Medication use and disability among migraineurs: a national probability sample. *Headache* 1992;32:223–8

11. Welch KM. Relationship of stroke and migraine. *Neurology* 1994;44:S33–6

12. Carolei A, Marini C, De Matteis G. History of migraine and risk of cerebral ischaemia in young adults. The Italian National Research Council Study Group on Stroke in the Young. *Lancet* 1996;347:1503–6

13. Ottman R, Lipton RB. Is the comorbidity of epilepsy and migraine due to a shared genetic susceptibility? *Neurology* 1996;47:918–24

14. Stewart WF, Shechter A, Liberman J. Physician consultation for headache pain and history of panic: results from a population-based study. *Am J Med* 1992;92:35S–40S

15. Merikangas KR, Angst J, Isler H. Migraine and psychopathology. Results of the Zurich cohort study of young adults. *Arch Gen Psychiatry* 1990;47:849–53

16. Breslau N, Davis GC. Migraine, major depression and panic disorder: a prospective epidemiologic study of young adults. *Cephalalgia* 1992;12:85–9

17. Brandt J, Celentano D, Stewart WF, *et al*. Personality and emotional disorder in a community sample of migraine headache sufferers. *Am J Psychiatry* 1990;147:303–8

18. Mathew NT. Transformed migraine. *Cephalalgia* 1993;13:78–83

19. Peres MFP, Young WB, Zukerman E, *et al*. Fibromyalgia is common in patients with transformed migraine. *Neurology* 2001;57:1326–8

CHAPTER 4

Pathophysiology of migraine

There are two main competing theories for migraine pathogenesis: the vasogenic theory and the neurogenic theory. At first these two theories appear to be at odds, but novel ways of looking at brain function indicate that they may complement each other.

THE VASOGENIC THEORY OF MIGRAINE

The premise of the vasogenic theory is that focal ischemia is the root cause of the migraine aura. Auras are due to hypoperfusion secondary to vasoconstriction of the blood vessel that supplies the cortical lobe corresponding to the aura symptom, be it visual, sensory or motor. Reactive vasodilation would explain the genesis of pain through stimulation of the perivascular pain-sensitive fibers. This theory would be in agreement with the throbbing quality of pain, its varied location and the pain relief caused by vasoconstrictive agents such as ergotamine. Patients undergoing the aura phase of their attacks were studied using ^{133}Xe blood flow techniques and these studies revealed a 17–35% reduction in cerebral blood flow in the posterior regions of the brain. More recent positron emission tomographic scan studies during the aura phase of migraine confirm these results and reveal slowly spreading hypoperfusion. Neither study showed evidence of ischemia.

THE NEUROGENIC THEORY OF MIGRAINE

The neurogenic theory has as its basis the cortical spreading depression of Leao (Figure 4.1). It predicts that alterations in blood flow develop as a consequence of neuronal events. During a migraine attack there is an initial brief hyperperfusion phase followed by a relatively sustained phase of hypoperfusion that corresponds to cortical spreading depression[1] (Figure 4.2). This probably reflects a wave of neuronal and glial depolarization followed by longer-lasting suppression of neural activity. Credence has been lent to this theory by recent magnetic resonance imaging studies using blood oxygenation level-dependent and perfusion-weighted imaging techniques during migraine with aura attacks, revealing signal changes characteristic of cortical spreading depression within the human brain[2]. These studies revealed an initial vasodilation occurring with the onset of visual aura that progressed contiguously over the occipital cortex at a rate of 3.5 ± 1.1 mm/min. This initial vasodilation was followed by hypoperfusion. The fact that the blood oxygenation level-dependent signal changes during aura abort at major sulci, that the light-evoked visual responses were suppressed during migraine with aura attacks and took 15 min to return to 80% of baseline, and that those areas first affected were the first to recover provides strong evidence consistent with the theory that an electrophysiologic event, such as cortical spreading depression (Figures 4.3 and 4.4), generates the migraine aura in the human visual cortex[2] (Figures 4.5–4.8).

THE TRIGEMINOVASCULAR SYSTEM

The brain is an insensate organ that lacks innervation by pain fibers. However, the dura mater and meningeal blood vessels are richly innervated by sensory nerve fibers that originate from the ophthalmic division of the trigeminal nerve. Together with the trigeminal nucleus they constitute the trigeminovascular system[3]. During a migraine attack these sensory fibers release vaso-dilating and permeability-promoting peptides from perivascular nerve endings, e.g. substance P, calcitonin gene-related peptide and neurokinin A. These peptides promote a sterile inflammatory response within the dura mater and cause the sensitization of sensory nerve fibers to previously innocuous stimuli (e.g. blood vessel pulsations or venous pressure changes) and manifest themselves as increased intracranial mechanosensitivity and hyperalgesia worsened by coughing or sudden head movement[4]. Calcitonin gene-related peptide levels have been found to be elevated in jugular venous blood during migraine attacks, returning to normal after administration of sumatriptan and amelioration of the headache. This is consistent with neuropeptide release from activated sensory nerves during the migraine attack and blockade of peptide release by sumatriptan, mediated via 5-HT$_{1B/1D}$ prejunctional receptors (Figure 4.9) on sensory terminals (Figure 4.10). A recent single photon emission computed tomography study provided the first direct evidence for the presence of plasma protein extravasation localized to extra-parenchymal regions ipsilateral to the side of pain during a spontaneous migraine attack.

Trigeminovascular activation occurs secondary to an initiation factor for migraine attacks. What initiates this is still unclear. Brainstem, cortical structures or neurochemical dysfunction may play an important role in either the genesis or modulation of migraines, or both. It now appears that the migraine brain is inherently more hyperexcitable either due to genetic factors (e.g. point mutations in genes encoding calcium channels, mitochondrial energy impairment and magnesium deficiency) or external factors (such as stress and hormonal changes).

Brainstem nuclei, including the periaqueductal gray matter, locus coeruleus and dorsal raphe nuclei (Figure 4.11), have been shown to either generate or suppress pain symptoms resembling migraine in animals and humans[5]. These locations in the brain stem do not seem to be activated as a response to head pain (Figure 4.12). Noradrenergic and serotoninergic nuclei participate in stress responses, anxiety and depressive states. Migraineurs may exhibit central hypersensitivity to dopaminergic stimulation, which has been linked to behaviors observed during migraine, such as yawning, irritability, hyperactivity, gastroparesis, nausea and vomiting. Molecular genetic studies have provided further evidence for the involvement of the dopaminergic system. Migraine is associated with the dopaminergic hypersensitivity phenotype and genes encoding the DRD$_2$ receptor[6].

The possibility of a 'migraine generator' in the rostral brainstem was raised by a positron emission tomography blood flow study performed during spontaneous unilateral headache in nine patients without aura[5]. Increased regional cerebral blood flow was found in medial brainstem predominantly contralateral to the headache, which persisted after relief of migraine pain with sumatriptan (Figure 4.13). Whether these brainstem nuclei serve as migraine generators or participate in modifying the threshold for neuronal activation or are part of the neuronal system that terminates an attack remains to be clarified (Figure 4.14).

REFERENCES

1. Cutrer FM, O'Donnell A, Sanchez DR. Functional neuroimaging: enhanced understanding of migraine pathophysiology. *Neurology* 2000;55:S36–45

2. Sanchez DR, Bakker D, Wu O, *et al.* Perfusion weighted imaging during migraine: spontaneous visual aura and headache. *Cephalalgia* 1999;19:701–7

3. Sanchez del Rio M, Moskowitz MA. The trigeminal system. In: Olesen J, Tfelt-Hansen P, Welch KM, eds. *The Headaches.* Philadelphia: Lippincott Williams & Wilkins, 2000:141–9

4. Moskowitz MA. The neurobiology of vascular head pain. *Ann Neurol* 1984;16:157–68

5. Weiller C, May A, Limmroth V, *et al.* Brain stem activation in spontaneous human migraine attacks. *Nat Med* 1995;1:658–60

6. Peroutka SJ, Price SC, Wilhoit TL, Jones KW. Comorbid migraine with aura, anxiety, and depression is associated with dopamine D2 receptor (DRD2) NcoI alleles. *Mol Med* 1998;4:14–21

CHAPTER 5

Migraine

Migraine is a common primary episodic headache disorder. In the United States, more than 17% of women and 6% of men had at least one migraine attack in the past year. Although the term migraine derives from the Greek word 'hemicrania', which means 'half of the head', it is not always a strictly unilateral headache; it can be bilateral and it is characterized by various combinations of neurologic, gastrointestinal and autonomic symptoms.

There are many migraine subtypes, including migraine without aura, migraine with aura, basilar migraine, familial hemiplegic migraine, status migrainosus and chronic (previously transformed) migraine.

According to the International Headache Society (IHS)'s classification and diagnostic criteria for primary headaches, certain clinical features must be present and organic disease must be excluded for headaches to qualify as migraine.

To diagnose migraine without aura, five attacks are needed, each lasting 4 to 72 h and having two of the following four characteristics: unilateral location, pulsating quality, moderate-to-severe intensity and aggravation by routine physical activity. In addition, the attacks must have at least one of the following: nausea (and/or vomiting) or photophobia and phonophobia.

Four phases of migraine (prodrome, aura, headache and postdrome) are recognized and may occur alone or in combination with any other phase. The prodrome consists of premonitory phenomena generally occurring hours to days before the headache and include mental and mood changes (depression, anger, euphoria), stiff neck, fatigue, yawning, food cravings, fluid retention and increase in urination.

The aura is composed of focal, neurologic symptoms that usually precede the headache, lasting in general less than 60 min. Visual symptoms are the most common, such as zigzag or scintilating figures (fortification spectrum), scotomata and distortions in shape and size. Motor, sensory or brainstem disturbances can also occur (Figures 5.1–5.9).

The headache phase is typically characterized by unilateral pain that is throbbing, moderate to marked in severity and aggravated by physical activity. The pain of migraine is invariably accompanied by other features. Nausea occurs in almost 90% of patients, while vomiting occurs in about one-third of migraineurs. Many patients experience sensory hyperexcitability manifested by photophobia, phonophobia and osmophobia, and seek a dark, quiet room. Other systemic symptoms, including anorexia, blurry vision, diarrhea, abdominal cramps, polyuria, pallor of the face, stiffness and tenderness of the neck and sweating, may also be noted during the headache phase. Impairment of concentration is common; less often there is memory impairment. Depression, fatigue, anxiety, nervousness and irritability are also frequent. Lightheadedness, rather than true vertigo, and a feeling of faintness may occur.

In the postdrome phase, the pain wanes. Following the headache, the patient may feel tired, washed out, irritable and listless and may have impaired concentration, scalp tenderness or mood changes. Some people feel unusually refreshed or euphoric after an attack, while others note depression and malaise.

A number of mechanisms and theories have been proposed to explain the causes of migraine. The strong familial association and the early onset of the disorder suggest that there is an important genetic component, and migraine has been considered to be a chanellopathy.

The pain distribution suggests involvement of the trigeminal nerve, trigeminal activation resulting in the release of neuropeptides, producing neurogenic inflammation with increased vascular permeability, and dilation of blood vessels. This is the trigeminal vascular model proposed by Moskowitz[1] (Figures 5.10–5.14).

Muscle contraction and tenderness might be another important component in migraine patients. Neurotransmitters including serotonin, dopamine, norepinephrine, glutamate, nitric oxide, GABA and other substances such as magnesium and melatonin have also been considered in migraine pathophysiology.

The goals of migraine treatment are to relieve or prevent the pain and associated symptoms of migraine and to optimize the patient's ability to function normally. To achieve these goals patients must learn to identify and avoid headache triggers. Pharmacologic treatment of migraine may be acute (abortive, symptomatic) or preventive (prophylactic). Patients experiencing frequent, severe headaches often require both approaches. The choice of treatment should be guided by the presence of comorbid conditions. A concurrent illness should be treated with a single agent when possible and agents that might aggravate a comorbid illness should be avoided. Biofeedback, relaxation techniques and other behavioral interventions can also be used as adjunctive therapy.

Many medications have been used for acute migraine treatment, including analgesics, antiemetics, anxiolytics, nonsteroidal anti-inflammatory drugs, ergots (Figure 5.15), steroids, major tranquilizers and narcotics. Recently, triptans (selective $5\text{-HT}_{1B/D}$ (serotonin) agonists; Figure 5.16) have been used with success (e.g. sumatriptan, rizatriptan, zolmitriptan and naratriptan).

Preventive treatments include a broad range of medications, most notably antidepressants, anticonvulsants, serotonin antagonists, β-blockers and calcium channel blockers.

CHAPTER 6

Trigeminal-autonomic cephalgias

INTRODUCTION

This chapter will discuss the distinct headache disorders known as the trigeminal-autonomic cephalgias (TACs). This group of primary headaches is characterized by short-duration unilateral head pains and associated ipsilateral autonomic symptoms. Recognized TACs include cluster headaches, chronic paroxysmal hemicrania (CPH), episodic paroxysmal hemicrania (EPH) and the syndrome of short-lasting unilateral neuralgiform headache with conjunctival injection and tearing (SUNCT); see Table 6.1. Cluster headaches are a fairly common condition while CPH and SUNCT may never be seen by physicians in their entire practice lifetime. What sets these headaches apart from the other primary headache disorders such as

migraine and tension-type headache is the extreme intensity of the headache and the unique associated symptoms representing both parasympathetic nervous system activation (eye lacrimation, conjunctival injection, nasal congestion or rhinorrhea) and sympathetic nervous system dysfunction (miosis, ptosis, partial Horner's syndrome). What distinguishes each of the TACs from each other is the duration of the headache attacks. SUNCT has the shortest attacks lasting 5 to 250 s (Figure 6.1), with CPH lasting 2 to 45 min (Figure 6.2) and cluster headaches lasting 15 to 180 min (Figure 6.3). What ties the syndromes together is a linkage between headache and autonomic symptoms. This clinical phenotype can be explained by an underlying trigeminal-autonomic reflex pathway which consists of a brainstem connection between

Table 6.1 The differential diagnosis for cluster headache involves the other known trigeminal-autonomic cephalgias: SUNCT, CPH, EPH, idiopathic stabbing headache and trigeminal neuralgia. Based on individual attack duration, attack frequency and associated symptoms, a correct diagnosis of cluster can be made. In the United States it takes an average of 6 years before a cluster patient is correctly diagnosed. It should not be difficult to make a diagnosis of cluster if a good headache history is taken. PPT, precipitant. Reproduced with permission from reference 1

Feature	Cluster	CPH	EPH	SUNCT	Stabbing headache	Trigeminal neuralgia
Gender (M:F)	4:1	1:3	1:1	2.3:1	F > M	F > M
Attack duration	15–18 min	2–45 min	1–30 min	5–250 s	<1 s	<1 s
Attack frequency	1–8/day	1–40/day	3–30/day	1/day–30/h	Few–many	Few–many
Autonomic features	+	+	+	+	−	−
Alcohol PPT	+	+	+	+	−	−
Indomethacin effect	+/−	+	+	−	+	−

the trigeminal nerve and the facial nerve (the site of the cranial parasympathetic outflow system). It is very important for the clinician to recognize the TACs as distinct headache disorders outside of migraine and tension-type headache, because treatment strategies are different for each headache. For example, CPH is an indomethacin-responsive headache syndrome, while cluster headaches and SUNCT do not respond to this non-steroidal anti-inflammatory agent. In the following paragraphs short descriptions of the distinct TACs will be given, following which a pictorial presentation of the TACs will be made including images on epidemiology, pathogenesis, clinical characteristics and treatment strategies (Figures 6.1–6.35).

CLUSTER HEADACHES

There is no more severe pain than that sustained by a cluster headache sufferer. Cluster headache is known as the 'suicide headache' (for other names of this condition, see Table 6.2), and if not for the rather short duration of attacks most cluster sufferers would choose death rather than continue suffering. Cluster headache is a primary headache syndrome (Figure 6.4). It is very stereotyped in its presentation and fairly easy to diagnose with an in-depth headache history. Fortunately cluster headaches are easy to treat in most individuals if the correct medications are used and the correct dosages are given. Our understanding of the pathogenesis of cluster headaches is increasing and with this there should arise better and more specific cluster therapies. Recently Klapper et al.[2] determined that the average time it takes for a cluster sufferer to be diagnosed correctly by the medical profession is 6.6 years. This statistic is unacceptable based on the pain and suffering cluster patients must endure when they are not treated correctly or not treated at all. In many instances cluster headache is misdiagnosed as migraine or sinus headache, so an inappropriate therapy regime is prescribed. The International Headache Society (IHS) in 1988 composed diagnostic criteria for cluster headache[3] (Table 6.3). Patients with cluster headache should experience at least 5 attacks of severe unilateral, orbital, supraorbital and/or temporal pain that lasts

Table 6.2 Cluster headache has been recognized in the literature by many names, some of which are still used today

Hemicrania angioparalytica (Eulenberg, 1878)
Sluder's sphenopalatine neuralgia (Sluder, 1908)
Ciliary neuralgia, migrainous neuralgia (Harris, 1926)
Autonomic faciocephalalgia (Brickner and Riley, 1935)
Erythromelalgia of the head, histaminic cephalalgia
   (Horton, 1939, 1941; Figure 6.10)

Table 6.3 International Headache Society's classification of cluster headache. Adapted with permission from reference 3

(1) At least five attacks fulfilling (2)–(4)
(2) Severe unilateral, orbital, supraorbital and/or temporal pain lasting 15 to 180 min untreated
(3) Headache is associated with at least one of the following signs that have to be present on the pain side:
    (a) conjunctival injection
    (b) lacrimation
    (c) nasal congestion
    (d) rhinorrhea
    (e) forehead and facial sweating
    (f) miosis
    (g) ptosis
    (h) eyelid edema
(4) Frequency of attacks: from one every other day to eight a day

Table 6.4 Distribution of associated symptoms with cluster headaches. Lacrimation is the most common symptom. Cluster patients do get 'migrainous associated symptoms'. If a cluster patient has typical cluster symptoms but also has nausea and vomiting, the diagnosis is still cluster and not migraine

Autonomic symptoms
Lacrimation (73%)
Conjunctival injection (60%)
Nasal congestion (42%)
Rhinorrhea (22%)
Partial Horner's syndrome (16–84%)

General symptoms
Nausea (10–54%; 29%)
Vomiting (1–15%; 9%)
Photophobia (5–72%)
Phonophobia (12–39%)

from 15 to 180 min untreated. The headache needs to be associated with at least one of the following signs or symptoms: lacrimation, conjunctival injection, rhinorrhea, nasal congestion, forehead and facial sweating, miosis, ptosis or eyelid edema (Table 6.4). Cluster headaches are typically side-fixed and will remain on the same side of the head for a patient's entire lifetime. Only 15% of

Table 6.5 Comparison chart looking at percentage of patients with migrainous symptoms (photophobia, phonophobia, nausea, vomiting) from three cluster investigations and the average percentage of these symptoms from seven migraine studies. Cluster patients have just as much photophobia and phonophobia as migraine patients but less nausea and vomiting. Photophobia and phonophobia should not be considered good differentiating symptoms between cluster and migraine. Data derived from Rozen TD, Niknam RM, Shechter AL, *et al. J Neurol Neurosurg Psychiatr* 2001;70:613–7; Nappi G, Micieli G, Cavallini A, *et al. Cephalalgia* 1992;12:165–8; Vingen JV, Pareja JA, Sovner LJ. *Cephalalgia* 1998;18:250–6. n/a, data not available

Symptom	Rozen, 2001	Nappi, 1992	Vingen, 1998	Migraine (n = seven studies)
Photophobia	80%	56%	91%	79%
Phonophobia	50%	15%	89%	80%
Nausea	53%	41%	n/a	87%
Vomiting	32%	24%	n/a	56%

patients will have a shift of sides between cluster periods. The pain of cluster headaches is described as sharp or boring and usually localizes behind the eye. During a cluster attack, cluster patients cannot and do not want to remain still. They typically pace the floors or even bang their heads against the wall to try and alleviate their pain. Cluster headaches are short in duration compared to some of the other primary headaches, usually with an average duration of 45 min to 1 h (Figure 6.3). Cluster patients will frequently have between one and three attacks per day. The headaches have a predilection for the first REM sleep phase, so the cluster patient will awaken with a severe headache 60 to 90 min after falling asleep (Figure 6.5). Cluster headaches can be of an episodic (greater than 14 headache-free days per year) or chronic (occuring for more than 1 year without remission or with < 14 headache-free days per year) subtype. Between 80–90% of cluster patients have the episodic variety (Figure 6.6). Cluster periods, or the time when patients are experiencing daily cluster attacks, usually last between 2 and 12 weeks and patients can have 1–2 cluster periods per year (Figure 6.7). It is not uncommon for a patient to experience a cluster period at the same time each year. This circadian periodicity suggests a hypothalamic generator for cluster headaches (Figures 6.8–6.9). In regard to age of onset, cluster headaches are a disorder of young people but the headaches do not start as young as they do in migraine. Typically cluster headaches will begin in the twenties or thirties, although they can start in the teens or even younger. Men appear to have one age peak of cluster onset in their twenties (Figure 6.11a), while women have one peak in their late teens and twenties and a second in their fifties or sixties (Figure 6.11b). In most instances cluster headaches should be easy to distinguish from migraine based upon the duration of individual attacks (cluster headaches last 15 min to 3 h versus migraines which last > 4 h) and the number of attacks experienced per day (cluster: one or more; migraine: none or one). In addition, only about 3% of cluster patients can remain still during a headache, while almost all migraineurs want to lie down with a migraine. It used to be thought that cluster patients did not experience 'migrainous symptoms' (nausea, vomiting, photophobia, phonophobia) and that these were good distinguishing characteristics between the two disorders, but this may not be true. Photophobia and phonophobia occur almost as frequently in cluster headaches as they do in migraine. Nausea and vomiting also occur in cluster patients, specifically females, but not nearly as frequently as in migraine (Table 6.5). With regard to the autonomic symptoms which are hallmarks of cluster attacks, only about 20% of migraineurs have associated ptosis, unilateral lacrimation or nasal congestion/rhinorrhea with their headaches. In addition, aura, which was supposed to be a migraine-only event, has now been shown to occur with cluster headaches, so the presence of aura cannot define a primary headache syndrome. Finally, migraine is a disorder of women and cluster headache is supposed to be a disorder of men (Figure 6.12). It is not uncommon for physicians to give a woman a

Table 6.6 Data illustrating how the male:female cluster headache gender ratio is decreasing over time. The cause of this is unknown but may reflect a true increase in cluster incidence or better diagnoses by physicians. In total, 482 patients (374 males, 108 females) were evaluated. Reproduced with permission from reference 4

Male to female ratios
Before 1960 6.2:1
1960–1969 5.6:1
1970–1979 4.3:1
1980–1989 3.0:1
1990–1995 2.1:1
Is this due to a decrease in male cluster patients or an
    increase in females, or better diagnosis?

Table 6.7 Abortive treatment of cluster headache. Sumatriptan injectable can provide relief within 5 min (Figure 6.13, Table 6.9). Oxygen is safe in all cluster patients, even those with cardiovascular risk factors (see also Table 6.8). Reproduced with permission from reference 1

High efficacy
    O_2
    sumatriptan subcutaneous (6 mg)
    IV/IM/SQ dihydroergotamine mesylate 0.5–1.0 mg
Limited efficacy
    zolmitriptan 5–10 mg oral
    ergotamine 1–2 mg oral or suppository
    intranasal lidocaine

Table 6.8 Oxygen is effective in up to 70% of cluster patients. A non-rebreather face mask should be used as delivery system. Reproduced with permission from reference 1

100% O_2 7–10 liters/min for 15 min
Efficacy 70% at 15 min
Most effective when headache is at maximum intensity
May delay rather than completely abort attack
Main limitation is accessibility

diagnosis of migraine even though she has typical cluster features just because she is a woman, falsely believing that women do not get cluster headaches. Cluster headaches undoubtedly occur in women, and there is a recent epidemiologic study from Italy suggesting that more women are developing or being diagnosed with cluster headaches (Table 6.6). The previous male:female cluster ratio of 6–7:1 has decreased to 2:1 in the 1990s. Female cluster headaches can appear exactly like male cluster headaches except that female cluster patients develop more nausea and vomiting with cluster attacks and have less miosis and ptosis than their male counterparts.

Table 6.9 Sumatriptan injectable is the fastest and most effective therapy for cluster headache at the present time. It is contraindicated in cluster patients with cardiovascular risk factors. Reproduced with permission from reference 1

Effective in 90% of patients for 90% of their attacks for both episodic and chronic cluster headache
Efficacy within 15 min in 50–75%
No tachyphylaxis
Attack frequency not increased with prolonged use
Not effective for cluster prophylaxis

Table 6.10 Surgical procedures for cluster headache are directed towards the sensory trigeminal nerve or cranial parasympathetic system (Figure 6.14). Surgery should only be considered once a patient is deemed refractory to medical treatment. Cluster patients who have only had one side of the head affected can get surgery in contrast to those who have had side-switching, as the latter are at great risk of having the headache switch sides after surgery

Procedures directed towards the sensory trigeminal nerve
    Alcohol injection into supraorbital and infraorbital nerves
    Alcohol injection into Gasserian ganglion
    Avulsion of infraorbital/supraorbital/supratrochlear nerves
    Retrogasserian glycerol injection (less corneal anesthesia)
    Radiofrequency trigeminal gangliorhyzolysis (75% effective,
        20% recurrence)
    Trigeminal root section
Procedures directed at autonomic pathways
    Section of greater superficial petrosal nerve
    Section of nervus intermedius

SUNCT

The syndrome of short-lasting unilateral neuralgiform headache attacks with conjunctival injection and tearing, or SUNCT, was first described by Sjaastad *et al.* in 1978 in an article entitled 'Multiple neuralgiform unilateral headache attacks associated with conjunctival injection and appearing in clusters'. The description of the complete syndrome came in 1989[5]. SUNCT is the rarest of the primary headache disorders with less than 30 documented cases. Many headache specialists have stated that they have never seen SUNCT and some still question the validity of the syndrome. SUNCT is comprised of brief attacks of moderate to severe head pain with associated autonomic disturbances of conjunctival injection, tearing, rhinorrhea or nasal obstruction (Table 6.11). The typical age of onset is between 40 and 70 years (Figure 6.15). SUNCT pain is normally localized to an orbital or periorbital distribution, although

Table 6.11 Proposed criteria for SUNCT syndrome. Reproduced from reference 6, with permission of Oxford University Press

Diagnostic criteria
(1) At least 30 attacks fulfilling (2)–(5)
(2) Attacks of unilateral, moderately severe, orbital or temporal stabbing or throbbing pain lasting from 15–120 s
(3) Attack frequency from 3 to 100/day
(4) Pain is associated with at least one of the following signs or symptoms of the affected side with feature (a) being most often present and very prominent:
    (a) conjunctival injection
    (b) lacrimation
    (c) nasal congestion
    (d) rhinorrhea
    (e) ptosis
    (f) eyelid edema
(5) At least one of the following:
    (a) There is no suggestion of one of the disorders listed in groups 5–11 (see Figure 2.1).
    (b) Such a disorder is suggested but excluded by appropriate investigations.
    (c) Such a disorder is present, but the first headache attacks do not occur in close temporal relation to the disorder.

Clinical note: The literature suggests that the most common secondary cause of SUNCT would be a lesion in the posterior fossa.

Table 6.12 SUNCT attacks are marked by associated symptoms of parasympathetic activation (lacrimation, conjunctival injection) and much less common sympathetic dysfunction (ptosis); *symptomatic side; **symptomatic cases; †one patient reported bilateral nasal stenosis during attacks; ††reported as being bilateral by one patient. Reproduced with permission from reference 7

	n
Lacrimation*	21 (2**)
Conjunctival injection*	20 (2**)
Rhinorrhea*	14 (1**)
Nasal obstruction*†	14 (1**)
Eyelid edema*	8 (1**)
Decreased palpebral fissure*	5 (1**)
Facial redness*	4 (1**)
Tachypnea, clinically observable	3
Photophobia*	2
Blepharospasm††	2
Miosis*	1
Feeling of facial sweating	1
Nausea	1
Ptosis	1
Feeling of foreign body in the eye*	1
Polyuria	1
Unpleasant feeling, nose	1
Dilated vessels, eyelids*	1

the forehead and temple can be the main site of pain (Figure 6.16). Head pain can radiate to the temple, nose, cheek, ear and palate. The pain is normally side-locked and remains unilateral throughout an entire attack. In rare instances SUNCT pain can be bilateral. Pain severity is normally moderate to severe, unlike cluster headache pain which is always severe. The pain is described most often as a stabbing, burning, pricking or electric shock-like sensation. Pain duration is extremely short, lasting between 5 and 250 s, with an average duration of 10 to 60 s (Figure 6.1). It is this extremely brief pain duration that sets SUNCT apart from other primary headache syndromes; SUNCT pain normally plateaus at a maximum intensity for several seconds and then quickly abates. SUNCT can occur at any time of the day, and does not show a tendency towards nocturnal attacks; only 1.2% of reported sufferers have night-time episodes (Figure 6.17). Attack frequency varies greatly between sufferers and within an individual sufferer. The usual attack frequency ranges anywhere from 1 to more than

80 episodes a day. Individuals can experience fewer than one attack an hour to more than 30. Mean attack frequency is 28 attacks per day. SUNCT is an episodic disorder that presents in a relapsing/remitting pattern. Each symptomatic period can last from several days to several months, and a person with SUNCT will typically have 1 to 2 symptomatic periods a year. The longest documented symptomatic period is 5 years, and the highest number of reported SUNCT episodes in one year is 22. Remissions typically last months but can last years. Symptomatic periods appear to increase in frequency and duration over time. All documented SUNCT patients experience conjunctival injection and lacrimation (ipsilateral to the side of the head pain) with each attack. Ipsilateral rhinorrhea and/or nasal obstruction occur in 67% of individuals. Less frequent associated symptoms include eyelid edema, a decreased palpebral fissure, facial redness, photophobia and blepharospasm (Table 6.12). Typically, conjunctival injection and eye tearing will start within 1 to 2 s of pain onset and remain until the head pain ceases, sometimes outlasting the pain by up to

Table 6.13 All patients with SUNCT must have an MRI to rule out secondary causes, especially vascular malformation in the cerebellopontine region. MRI ($n = 12$), CT ($n = 11$), angiography ($n = 6$); *symptomatic side, **symptomatic cases. Reproduced with permission from reference 7

Patient	Procedure	Results
2	CT	Some enlarged sulci in frontal area
3	CT, MRI	Cholesteatoma*
5	MRI	Bilateral lacunar infarcts
7		
18	Head x-ray	Osteoma in anterior part of scalp
20**	MRI, angiography	Vascular malformation in cerebellopontine region*
21**		

Table 6.14 Until recently multiple medications had been tried in SUNCT, all without success. Recently several case reports have documented the efficacy of lamotrigine, gabapentin and topiramate for SUNCT; –, treatment had no effect; x, treatment worsened condition; SC, subcutaneous; IV, intravenous; *one patient with slight improvement. Reproduced from reference 6, with permission of Oxford University Press

Treatment	Dosage (max/day)	Response	n
Pharmacologic			
Aspirin	1800 mg	–	6
Paracetamol	4 g	–	6
Indomethacin	200 mg	–	9
Naproxen	1 g	–	3
Ibuprofen	1200 mg	–	3
Ergotamine (oral)	3 mg	–	7
Dihydroergotamine (IV)	3 mg	–	1
Sumatriptan (oral)	300 mg	–*	5
Sumatriptan (SC)	6 mg	–	1
Prednisone (oral)	100 mg	–	7
Methysergide	8 mg	–	4
Verapamil	480 mg	x	5
Valproate	1500 mg	–*	5
Lithium	900 mg	–	3
Propranolol	160 mg	–	3
Amitriptyline	100 mg	–	2
Carbamazepine	1200 mg	–	10
Procedures or infusions			
Lignocaine (IV)	4 mg/min	–	2
Greater occipital nerve	block	–	4

30 s. Rhinorrhea, on the other hand, starts in the mid-to-late phase of an attack. Nausea, vomiting, photophobia and phonophobia are not normally associated with SUNCT. SUNCT can arise spontaneously, but many sufferers have identified triggering maneuvers, including mastication, nose blowing, coughing, forehead touching, eyelid squeezing, neck movements (rotation, extension and flexion) and ice cream eating. In SUNCT there is no refractory period between pain attacks, so that if a trigger zone is stimulated during the ending phase of a previous attack, a new one can begin immediately. This is unlike the refractory period of trigeminal neuralgia. The true epidemiology of SUNCT is not known, and there is no prevalence or incidence data available. The extremely low number of reported cases suggests it is a very rare syndrome. All patients with SUNCT must have an MRI to rule out secondary causes (Table 6.13). SUNCT does appear to have a clear male predominance, with a male:female ratio of 4.25:1[6]. SUNCT is a disease of middle-aged

Table 6.15 Chronic paroxysmal hemicrania (CPH) is a relatively rare condition even in headache specialty clinics. By 1989, 84 cases had been described in the literature. CPH case reports are no longer published because this syndrome is now recognized as a true primary headache disorder. Reproduced with permission from reference 9

Published case reports	Year	n
Sjaastad & Dale	1974	2
Sjaastad & Dale	1976	1
Kayed et al.	1978	1
Price & Posner	1978	1
Christoffersen	1979	1
Manzoni & Terzano	1979	1
Leblanc et al.	1980	1
Sjaastad et al.	1980	2
Stein & Rogado	1980	2
Guerra	1981	2
Hochman	1981	1
Manzoni et al.	1981	1
Rapoport et al.	1981	1
Jensen et al.	1982	1
Kilpatrick & King	1982	2
Pelz & Meskey	1982	1
Geaney	1983	1
Peatty & Clifford Rose	1983	1
Thevenet et al.	1983	3
Bogucki et al.	1984	2
Boulliat	1984	1
Dutta	1984	1
Pfaffenrath et al.	1984	4
Pradalier & Dry	1984	1
Sjaastad et al.	1984	2
Drummond	1985	1
Granella et al.	1985	3
Heckl	1986	2
Pollman & Pfaffenrath	1986	1
Bogucki & Kozubski	1987	1
Centonze et al.	1987	3
Durko & Klimek	1987	1
Hannerz et al.	1987	1
Joubert et al.	1987	1
Kudrow et al.	1987	6
Nebudova	1987	1
Rasmussen	1987	4
Pearce et al.	1987	1
	Sum:	63
Unpublished case reports		
Bousser		2
Davalos		1
Graham		1
Greene		1
Jaeger		2
Manzoni		1
Mathew		2
Nappi		2
Sjaastad		8
Wall		1
	Sum:	21
	Total:	84

Table 6.16 Proposed criteria for chronic paroxysmal hemicrania and episodic paroxysmal hemicrania. Reproduced from reference 6, with permission of Oxford University Press

Chronic paroxysmal hemicrania
Diagnostic criteria

(1) At least 30 attacks fulfilling (2)–(5)
(2) Attacks of severe unilateral, orbital, supraorbital and/or temporal pain always on the same side lasting 2–45 min
(3) Attack frequency above five a day for more than half the time (periods with lower frequency may occur)
(4) Pain is associated with at least one of the following signs/symptoms on the pain side:

    (a) conjunctival injection
    (b) lacrimation
    (c) nasal congestion
    (d) rhinorrhea
    (e) ptosis
    (f) eyelid edema

(5) At least one of the following:

    (a) There is no suggestion of one of the disorders listed in groups 5–11 (see Figure 2.1).
    (b) Such a disorder is suggested but excluded by appropriate investigations.
    (c) Such a disorder is present, but the first headache attacks do not occur in close temporal relation to the disorder.

Note: Most cases respond rapidly and absolutely to indomethacin (usually in doses of 150 mg/day or less)

Episodic paroxysmal hemicrania
Diagnostic criteria

(1) At least 30 attacks fulfilling (2)–(6)
(2) Attacks of severe unilateral, orbital or temporal pain, or both, that is always unilateral and lasts from 1–30 min
(3) An attack frequency of three or more a day
(4) Clear intervals between bouts of attacks that may last from months to years
(5) Pain is associated with at least one of the following signs or symptoms on the painful side:

    (a) conjunctival injection
    (b) lacrimation
    (c) nasal congestion
    (d) rhinorrhea
    (e) ptosis
    (f) eyelid edema

(6) At least one of the following:

    1. There is no suggestion of one of the disorders listed in groups 5–11 (see Figure 2.1).
    2. Such a disorder is suggested but excluded by appropriate investigations.
    3. Such a disorder is present, but the first headache attacks do not occur in close temporal relation to the disorder.

Note: In most cases responds rapidly and absolutely to indomethacin (usually 150 mg/day or less)

and older individuals with no reported cases below age 23. Up until recently there have been no reported therapies for SUNCT (Table 6.14), although several case reports documenting relief with lamotrigine and topiramate have come into the literature.

CHRONIC PAROXYSMAL HEMICRANIA

Chronic paroxysmal hemicrania is a very rare headache syndrome first described by Sjaastad and Dale in 1974[8] (Table 6.15; for proposed criteria of this condition see Table 6.16). Unlike cluster headaches and SUNCT, CPH has a female predominance, with a female:male ratio of 3:1. CPH normally develops in the second or third decade of life but it can occur at any age (Figures 6.19 and 6.20). The natural history of this disorder is unknown (Figure 6.21). Clinically CPH patients have strictly unilateral headaches and the same side of the head is always affected. The pain location is normally orbital, temporal and above or behind the ear. The pain is very severe and is described as boring or claw-like (Figure 6.22). Attacks are short-lasting, between 2 and 45 min (Figure 6.2). Individuals can have between 1 and 40 attacks in a day; median frequency is 5 to 10 attacks per day. Unlike cluster headache there is no predilection for nocturnal attacks, although CPH attacks can certainly awaken patients from sleep (Figure 6.23). In regard to associated symptoms, most CPH patients exhibit lacrimation (62%), followed by nasal congestion (42%), conjunctival injection and rhinorrhea (36%) and ptosis (33%) (Table 6.17). Neck movements and external pressure to the transverse processes of C4 to C5 or the C2 nerve root can trigger CPH attacks. In phenotype, CPH is characterized by short-duration and more frequent cluster attacks. Unlike cluster patients, CPH patients typically remain still during an attack and by definition CPH responds to indomethacin treatment (Table 6.16). It does not matter how many years a patient has suffered from CPH and how many therapies they have tried, once indomethacin is administered the headaches will be gone within 48 h and remain alleviated as long as the patient remains on indomethacin (Figure 6.33). Very few other

Table 6.17 Autonomic symptoms mark the chronic paroxysmal hemicrania syndrome, specifically those suggesting cranial parasympathetic activation. Reproduced with permission from reference 9

Symptoms and signs	n
Lacrimation	52
Nasal stenosis	35
Conjunctival injection	30
Rhinorrhea	30
Ptosis	28
Photophobia	18
Miosis	15
Nausea	12
Generalized sweating	8
VI hypersensitivity	7
Phonophobia	6
Temporal artery pulsation	5
Visual phenomena	4
Temporal artery dilatation	4
Tinnitus	3
Vomiting	2
V2 hypersensitivity	2
Exophthalmus	1

Table 6.18 Chronic paroxysmal hemicrania (CPH) is one of the indomethacin-responsive headache syndromes. When a CPH patient cannot tolerate indomethacin or has contraindications to this drug, there are very few, if any other, medications that work in this disorder. Reproduced with permission from reference 9

Drug	Partial efficacy reports	Total number of reports
Salicylates	25	37
Ergotamine	3	36
Prednisone	2	18
β-Receptor blocking agents	0	13
Pizotifen	0	11
Carbamazepine	0	11
Lithium	1	11
Amitriptyline	0	8
Ketoprofen	1	7
Methysergide	0	7
Butazolidin	1	6
Naproxen	4	5
Phenobarbital	0	5
Oxygen	0	4
Tiapride	0	3
Ibuprofen	0	3
Diclofenac	2	2
Valproate	0	1
Verapamil	0	1
Clonazepam	0	1
Nimodipine	0	1
Histamine	0	1
Placebo	0	7

medications have ever worked for patients with CPH (Table 6.18). Secondary causes of CPH reported in the literature include: gangliocytoma of the sella turcica, pancoast tumor, frontal lobe tumor and cavernous sinus menigioma.

Episodic paroxysmal hemicrania (EPH) is characterized by frequent daily attacks of unilateral short-duration headaches with associated autonomic symptoms. EPH is really CPH, except EPH has periods of headache remission lasting weeks or months (Table 6.16 and Figure 6.21). There is debate if EPH is just an episodic variant of CPH or its own entity. Attack duration in EPH varies from 1 to 30 min with attack frequency between 6 and 30 individual headaches per day. EPH unlike CPH may not have a gender predominance. EPH like CPH invariably responds to indomethacin. There are reports in the literature of transformation from EPH to CPH suggesting these two conditions are ends of a spectrum.

REFERENCES

1. American Headache Society. Neurology Ambassador Program. http://www.ahsnet.org/ambass/ 3/27/2002
2. Klapper JA, Klapper A, Voss T. The misdiagnosis of cluster headache: a nonclinic, population-based Internet survey. *Headache* 2000;40:730–5
3. Headache Classification Committee of the International Headache Society. Classification and diagnostic criteria for headache disorders, cranial neuralgias and facial pain. *Cephalalgia* 1988;8 (Suppl 7):1–96
4. Manzoni GC. Male preponderance of cluster headache progressively decreasing over the years. *Headache* 1997;35:588–9
5. Sjaastad O, Saunte C, Salvesen R, *et al.* Shortlasting unilateral neuralgiform headache attacks with conjunctival injection, tearing, sweating, and rhinorrhea. *Cephalalgia* 1989;9:147–56
6. Goadsby PJ, Lipton RB. A review of paroxysmal hemicranias, SUNCT syndrome and other short-lasting headaches with automatic feature, including new cases. *Brain* 1997;120:193–209
7. Pareja JA, Sjaastad O. SUNCT syndrome. A clinical review. *Headache* 1997;37:195–202
8. Sjaastad O, Dale I. Evidence for a new, treatable headache entity. *Headache* 1997;14:105–8
9. Antonaci F, Sjaastad O. Chronic paroxysmal hemicrania (CPH): A review of the clinical manifestations. *Headache* 1989;29:648–56

CHAPTER 7

Tension-type headaches

INTRODUCTION

The most controversial and difficult boundary among primary headaches is the one between migraine and tension-type headache. While some view these disorders as distinct entities, others favor the 'spectrum' or 'continuum' concept, the idea that migraine and tension-type headache exist as polar ends on a continuum of severity, varying more in degree than in kind (Figure 7.1). Lipton et al.[1] in the 'spectrum' study found that migrainous and tension-type headaches in migraine patients responded to sumatriptan, supporting the spectrum theory. In the early phase of a migraine headache, the patient may have mild, non-pulsating pain and a lack of nausea, vomiting, photophobia and phonophobia, in which case the headache resembles a tension-type headache. Individuals often report only the symptoms of tension-type headache, yet have headaches that respond to migraine-specific treatment on prospective diary studies.

The International Headache Society (IHS) classification of headache, published in 1988, defined diagnostic criteria for primary headaches, including migraine and tension-type headaches (see Table 7.1). These criteria were more complete, explicit, and rigorous than criteria used in past studies, and led to an important advance in the research of headache disorders. However, tension-type headache was defined as recurrent headache without the features of migraine, perhaps artificially dividing a single disorder.

Table 7.1 IHS criteria for migraine and tension-type headache

Migraine
≥ 5 attacks lasting 4–72 h
Two of the following four:
  unilateral
  pulsating
  moderate to severe intensity
  aggravation by routine physical activity
One of the following:
  nausea and/or vomiting
  photophobia and phonophobia
No evidence on history or examination of disease that
  might cause headaches

Tension-type headache
10 attacks lasting 30 min–7 days
Two of the following four:
  bilateral
  not pulsating
  mild or moderate intensity
  no aggravation by routine physical activity
One of the following:
  no nausea/vomiting
  either photophobia or phonophobia or neither
No evidence on history or examination of disease that
  might cause headaches

Adapted with permission from reference 2

EPIDEMIOLOGY

Tension-type headache is the most common headache type. Estimates of its prevalence have varied widely. In Western countries, one-year prevalence ranges from 28–63% in men and from 34–86% in women, depending, in part, on methodologic differences between studies. A lifetime prevalence of 69% in men and 88% in women, and a one-year prevalence of 63% in men and 86% in women, was found in Denmark[3]. Interestingly, in mainland China there was a very low prevalence of tension-type headache[4].

The prevalence of chronic tension-type headache has varied from 2–3% in three Western studies[3,5].

PATHOPHYSIOLOGY

The term tension-type headache represents a compromise between those who believed this entity to be due to psychologic tension and those who felt muscle tension to be paramount. Ultimately, very little is known about the pathophysiology of tension-type headache. The IHS recognizes tension-type headache with and without a pericranial muscle disorder. Muscle tenderness may be seen in migraine, and findings in EMG and pressure algometry studies are inconsistent, even in the pericranial muscle abnormality group of tension-type headache patients.

IMPACT AND COSTS

Tension-type headaches often interfere with activities of daily living[6]. Eighteen percent of tension-type headache sufferers had to discontinue normal activity, while 44% experienced some limitation of function. Like migraine, tension-type headache is a disorder of middle life, striking individuals early in life and continuing to affect them through their peak productive years. All migraineurs, and 60% of tension-type headache patients, have a diminished capacity for work or other activities during an attack. In a Danish study, 43% of employed migraineurs and 12% of employed tension-type headache sufferers missed one or more days of work because of headache. Migraine caused at least one day of missed work for 5% of sufferers, while tension-type headache caused a day of missed work for 9%. Annually, per 1000 employed individuals, 270 lost work days were due to migraine and 820 were due to tension-type headache. Despite

prominent disability, nearly 50% of migraineurs and more than 80% of tension-type headache patients had never consulted their general practitioner because of headache[7]. Patients with daily headaches may have even more disability than episodic migraine and tension-type headache sufferers, although there are no data to confirm this assumption.

CONCLUSIONS

The pathophysiology of tension-type headache is not clearly understood. Raskin introduced the headache 'continuum' in 1988. In the last decade the pathogenesis of tension-type headache has again been called into question (Figure 7.2). Patients with migraine often suffer from milder headaches which meet the IHS criteria for tension-type headache[8,9]. These milder tension-type headaches seen in migraineurs often have a few associated migrainous features such as phonophobia or photophobia[10]. Cady et al.[11] observed that non-IHS migraine and tension-type headaches in patients with migraine respond to triptans, supporting theories of a common pathophysiology. Lipton et al.[1] demonstrated that in patients with migraine, sumatriptan was effective for their tension-type headaches (Figure 7.3). Tension-type headaches in patients with no migraine history seemingly lack migrainous features and do not respond to triptans[12,13]. To clarify these issues a prospective trial is needed testing triptans in migraineurs and non-migraineurs[14].

REFERENCES

1. Lipton RB, Stewart WF, Cady R, *et al.* 2000 Wolff Award. Sumatriptan for the range of headaches in migraine sufferers: results of the Spectrum Study. *Headache* 2000;40:783–91
2. Headache Classification Committee of the International Headache Society. Classification and diagnostic criteria for headache disorders, cranial neuralgias and facial pain. *Cephalalgia* 1988;8 (Suppl 7):1–96
3. Rasmussen BK, Jensen R, Schroll M, Olesen J. Epidemiology of headache in a general population – a prevalence study. *J Clin Epidemiol* 1991;44:1147–57

4. Wong TW, Wong KS, Yu TS, Kay R. Prevalence of migraine and other headaches in Hong Kong. *Neuroepidemiology* 1995;14:82–91

5. Castillo J, Munoz P, Guitera V, *et al*. Epidemiology of chronic daily headache in the general population. *Headache* 1999;39:190–6

6. Rasmussen BK. Epidemiology and socio-economic impact of headache. *Cephalalgia* 1999;19:20–3

7. Rasmussen BK, Olesen J. Symptomatic and nonsymptomatic headaches in a general population. *Neurology* 1992;42:1225–31

8. Rasmussen BK, Jensen R, Schroll M, Olesen J. Interrelations between migraine and tension-type headache in the general population. *Arch Neurol* 1992;49:914–8

9. Ulrich V, Russell MB, Jensen R, Olesen J. A comparison of tension-type headache in migraineurs and in non-migraineurs: a population-based study. *Pain* 1996;67:501–6

10. Iversen HK, Langemark M, Andersson PG, *et al*. Clinical characteristics of migraine and episodic tension-type headache in relation to old and new diagnostic criteria. *Headache* 1990;30:514–9

11. Cady RK, Gutterman D, Saiers JA, Beach ME. Responsiveness of non-IHS migraine and tension-type headache to sumatriptan. *Cephalalgia* 1997;17:588–90

12. Brennum J, Kjeldsen M, Olesen J. The 5-HT$_1$-like agonist sumatriptan has a significant effect in chronic tension-type headache. *Cephalalgia* 1992;12:375–9

13. Brennum J, Brinck T, Schriver L, *et al*. Sumatriptan has no clinically relevant effect in the treatment of episodic tension-type headache. *Eur J Neurol* 1996;3:23–8

14. Olesen J. Responsiveness of non-IHS migraine and tension-type headache to sumatriptan. *Cephalalgia* 1997;17:559

CHAPTER 8

Secondary headaches

The International Headache Society (IHS) has classified the secondary headaches into eight distinct categories based upon their causes (Figure 2.1). Secondary headaches can often have the same characteristics as primary headache disorders such as migraine and tension-type headache. Some of the secondary headaches can have serious and at times life-threatening causes. Fortunately, the vast majority of headache complaints are due to primary headache disorders such as migraine or tension-type headache. Many different diseases may present with the symptom of headache, and physicians must determine which cases need to be investigated further for possible secondary causes.

Not all headache patients need to be imaged; in fact the 'gold standard' in headache diagnosis is a complete and thorough history backed by a general physical and a neurologic examination. The primary purpose of radiographic investigation in headache patients is to exclude secondary causes in patients with unusual histories or abnormal physical exams. Certain clinical or historical features

should be considered 'red flags' and will warrant further diagnostic evaluation.

'Red flags' include: (i) a new sudden-onset headache in patients without previous headache or in patients who have cancer or test positive for HIV; (ii) the presence of new neurologic symptoms such as changes in vision, cognition or personality; (iii) precipitation of headache by strain or exertion; (iv) a change in headache pattern in a patient with a known headache disorder; (v) any new-onset headache after the age of 50; and (vi) headache accompanied by systemic symptoms such as fever, nuchal rigidity, jaw claudication and weight loss.

Symptomatic or secondary headaches have not been well described clinically, and studying secondary causes in a prospective manner offers many challenges. Analyzing secondary causes for headache will be important to elucidate potential mechanisms and locations involved in the primary disorders.

This chapter includes images of some of the secondary causes for headache (Figures 8.1–8.41).

Section II Headache Illustrated

List of Illustrations

Figure 6.12

Cluster predominantly occurs in men, although more women are being diagnosed with cluster headache

Figure 6.13

Reduction in pain severity after administration of sumatriptan injectable to patients with cluster headache

Figure 6.14

Presently the most effective surgical therapy for cluster is radiofrequency lesioning of the gasserian (trigeminal) ganglion

Figure 6.15

SUNCT is considered a disorder of the elderly, although there are some reported cases younger than age 40

Figure 6.16

SUNCT pain is located in or around the eye and/or the forehead region

Figure 6.17

SUNCT attacks tend to cluster around morning and afternoon/evening times, although attacks can occur at any time during the day

Figure 6.18

Orbital phlebogram showing narrowing of the superior ophthalmic vein and partial occlusion of the cavernous sinus in an episodic cluster patient

Figure 6.19

Chronic paroxysmal hemicrania typically starts to occur in the teens or twenties, very similar to the age of onset of cluster

Figure 6.20

Both females and males who develop chronic paroxysmal hemicrania typically have their first attacks in their teens or twenties

Figure 6.21

The natural history of chronic paroxysmal hemicrania is unknown

Figure 6.22

Quality of chronic paroxysmal hemicrania pain

Figure 6.23

Chronic paroxysmal hemicrania attacks, unlike cluster attacks, occur anytime during the day and night and do not have a predeliction for nocturnal attacks

Figure 6.24

Cluster is not considered to have a genetic predisposition as is seen in migraine, but first-degree relatives have a 14-fold increased risk of developing cluster headaches in their lifetime

Figure 6.25

Cluster headache has been linked to a typical facies, eye color and certain medical conditions

Figure 6.26

A comparison of trigeminovascular activation, cranial parasympathetic activation and sympathetic dysfunction

Figure 6.27

Changes in calcitonin gene-related peptide and vasoactive intestinal polypeptide levels during migraine, cluster and chronic paroxysmal hemicrania attacks

Figure 6.28

Dilation of the ophthalmic artery during a spontaneous cluster attack

Figure 6.29

Urine melatonin levels examined for up to 14 months in episodic cluster headache patients and healthy controls

Figure 6.30

Hypothalamic activation during a cluster attack on PET

Figure 6.31

Image showing how the hypothalamus, trigeminal sensory, cranial parasympathetic and carotid sympathetic systems interact to produce a cluster headache

Figure 6.32

Transition from episodic to chronic cluster and vice versa

Figure 6.33

Indomethacin is the sole treatment of choice in chronic paroxysmal hemicrania

Figure 6.34

Orbital phlebography in a 49-year-old man with SUNCT

Figure 6.35

BOLD contrast-MRI of the brain of a 71-year-old woman with SUNCT syndrome

Figure 7.1

'The continuum of benign recurring headache' by Raskin

Figure 7.2

Reclassification of headache diagnosis based on diary review

Figure 7.3

Pain-free response at 2 h by headache attack type in individuals with an initial diagnosis of tension-type headache and a final diagnosis of migraine

Figure 8.1

Vascular compresssion theory for trigeminal neuralgia

Figure 8.2

Overlapping pain referral patterns from myofascial trigger points in various masticatory and cervical muscles produce typical unilateral or bilateral migraine or tension-type headache

Figure 8.3

Referred pain from superficial masseter and upper trapezius myofascial trigger points may produce unilateral or bilateral tension-type and migraine headache symptoms

Figure 8.33

Twelve-year-old boy with two prior episodes of ophthalmoplegic migraine

Figure 8.34

Twenty-three-year-old woman with one prior episode of ophthalmoplegic migraine

Figure 8.35

Eight-year-old girl with one prior episode of spontaneously resolving oculomotor nerve palsy

Figure 8.36

Sixty-three-year-old female presents with right eye pain and ptosis

Figure 8.37

Elderly patient presents with complaint of recent memory difficulties, dizziness, headache and gait disturbances

Figure 8.38

Forty-year-old female presents with sudden-onset, right-sided headache with nausea and vomiting, decreased right facial sensation, dysarthria, partial pointing of right arm, ataxia, increased deep tendon reflexes and sensory loss in left hand

Figure 8.39

Seventy-year-old male presents with bilateral parietal headache and unsteady gait

Figure 8.40

Twenty-six-year-old male presents with severe headache and pulsatile tinnitus

Figure 8.41

Twenty-eight-year-old female with a history of Dandy–Walker syndrome diagnosed at age 16 presents with sudden onset headache

Illustrations

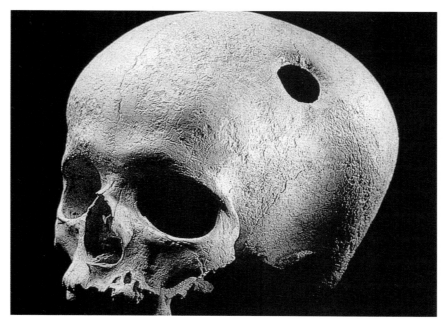

Figure 1.1 Trepanned skull, approximately 3000 years old. Of course, we do not know why this individual had trepanation. He did, however, survive long enough (this is 1000 BC) to generate new bone growth at the margin of the trepanned hole. Reproduced with kind permission of John Edmeads

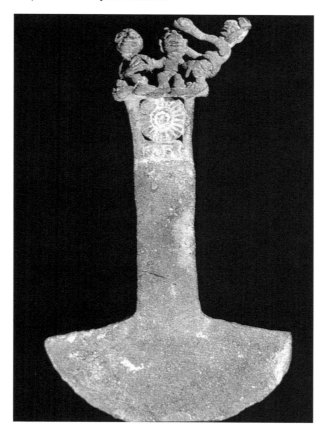

Figure 1.2 Trepanation has been done around the world. This is a tumi, a pre-Columbian trepan from Peru. Note the instructions for use on top of the handle. Reproduced with kind permission of John Edmeads

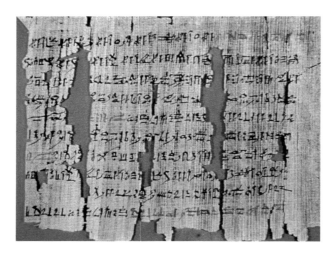

Figure 1.3 Papyrus from Thebes, Egypt (2500 BC). Now in a British museum. It is totally illegible, and therefore instantly recognizable as a prescription

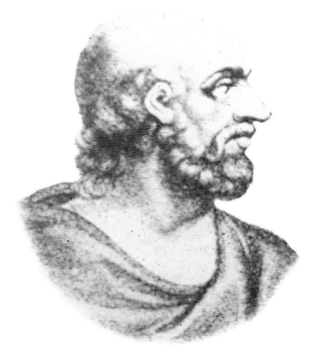

Figure 1.5 Hippocrates described migraine circa 400 BC. Courtesy of the National Library of Medicine, Bethesda, USA

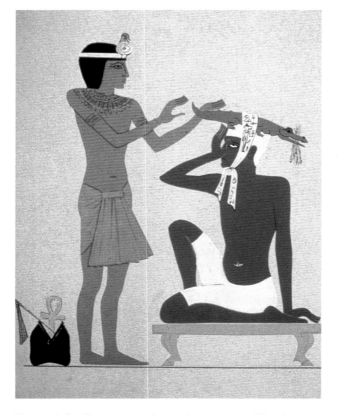

Figure 1.4 Cartoon, translating above papyrus: 'The physician shall take a crocodile made of clay, with sacred grain in its mouth, and an eye of faience. He shall bind it to the head of the patient with a strip of fine linen upon which is written the names of the Gods. And the physician shall pray'

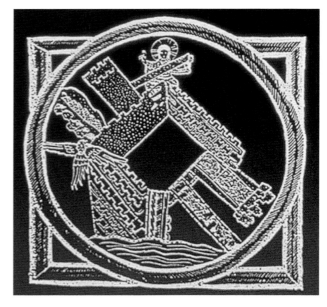

Figure 1.6 'Vision of the Heavenly City' from a manuscript of *Hildegard's Scivias* written at Bingen (circa 1180 AD)

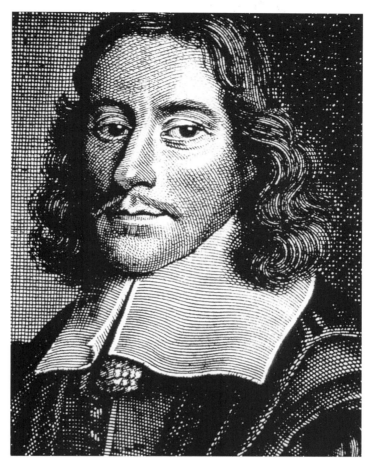

Figure 1.7 Thomas Willis, the father of neurology. The first to postulate that 'megrim' was due to blood 'estuating' (stagnating) in the dural vessels, distending them and producing head pain. Courtesy of the National Library of Medicine, Bethesda, USA

3. As to the differences of the Headach, the common diftinction is, That the pain of the Head is either without the Skull, or within its cavity : The former is a more rare and a more gentle difeafe, becaufe the parts above the Skull are not fo fenfible as the interior *Meninges*; nor are they watered with fo plentiful a flood of Blood, that by its fudden and vehement incurfion, they may be eafily diftended, or inflamed above meafure. Secondly, The other kind of Headach, to wit, within the Skull, is more frequent, and much more cruel, becaufe the Membranes, cloathing the Brain, are very fenfible, and the Blood is poured upon them by a manifold paffage, and by many and greater Arteries. Further, becaufe the Blood or its Serum, fometimes paffing thorow all the Arteries at once, both the *Carotides* and the *Vertebrals*, and fometimes apart, thorow thefe or thofe, on the one fide or the oppofite, bring hurt to the *Meninges*, hence the pain is caufed that is interior; which is either univerfal, infefting the whole Head or its greateft part; or particular, which is limited to fome private region; and fometimes produces a Meagrim on the fide, fometimes in the forepart, and fometimes in the hinder part of the Head.

Figure 1.8 Original publication of Thomas Willis' work, *The London Practice of Physick*. He stated that migraine was caused by vasodilation

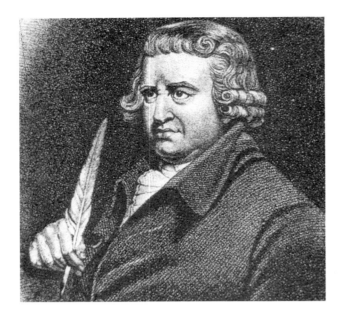

Figure 1.9 Erasmus Darwin, Charles' grandfather, a physician, lived in the eighteenth century. He postulated that since migraine, as Willis suggested, was due to too much blood in the head, ideal treatment would be to construct a giant centrifuge, put the patient in it and spin him. As the blood left the head, the headache should disappear. Fortunately, the technology was not available to mount the experiment. Courtesy of the National Library of Medicine, Bethesda, USA

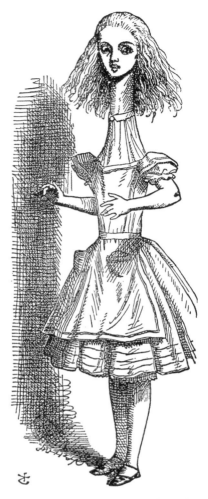

Figure 1.11 Illustration by John Tenniel from *Alice in Wonderland*. Was Lewis Carroll writing his migraine auras into his book?

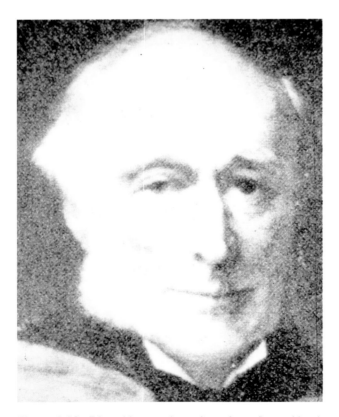

Figure 1.10 Edward Liveing, the author of an influential book on migraine from 1873, which argued that 'megrim' was a 'nerve-storm' or epileptic manifestation

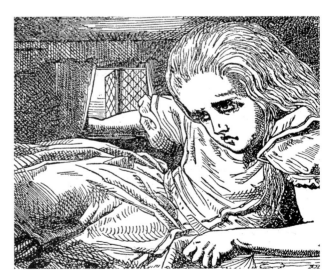

Figure 1.12 Illustration by John Tenniel from *Alice in Wonderland*. The image depicts the sense of being too large for one's surroundings

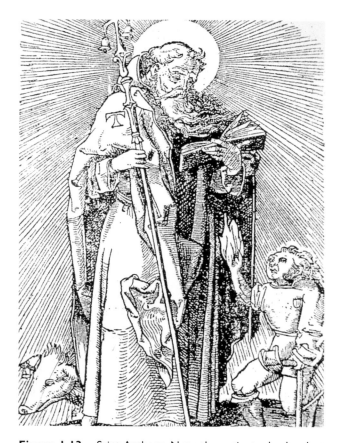

Figure 1.13 Saint Anthony. Note the patient who has lost limbs as a result of gangrene due to ergotism (eating bread made from rye contaminated with ergot fungus). Limbs turned black, as though charred by fire, then fell off. Hence the term 'St. Anthony's Fire'. If you prayed to Saint Anthony, your symptoms might improve. Note Anthony's pet pig. Courtesy of the National Library of Medicine, Bethesda, USA

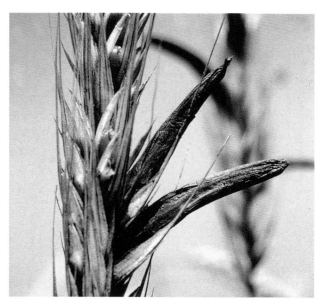

Figure 1.14 A stalk of grain upon which are growing two purple excrescences – *Claviceps purpurea,* or 'ergot fungus'. Reproduced with kind permission of John Edmeads

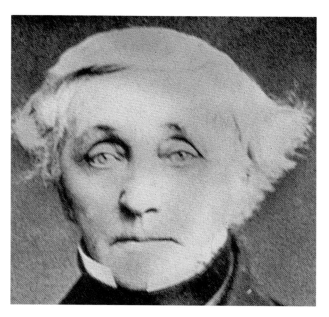

Figure 1.15 As the botanists argued over the nature of ergot, the chemists were attempting to unravel the mystery of its composition. Heinrich Wiggers, a pharmacist of Göttingen, Germany was probably the first to analyze ergot with the set purpose of trying to isolate the active principle or principles. In 1831 he tested his ergot extracts in animals. Among the models was the 'rooster comb test' – when fed ergotin the rooster became ataxic, nauseous, acquired a blanched comb and suffered from severe convulsions, dying days later. The rooster comb test continued to be used into the following century by investigators studying the physiologic properties of ergot

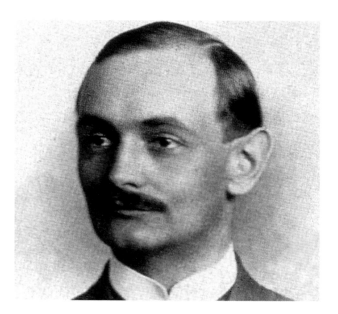

Figure 1.16 In 1918, Arthur Stroll, a young chemist working in Basel, Switzerland announced the isolation of the first pure crystalline substance, ergotamine. Professor Stroll made many additional contributions to our understanding of ergot, and in 1917 became the founder of the Sandoz 'Department of Pharmaceutical Specialities'

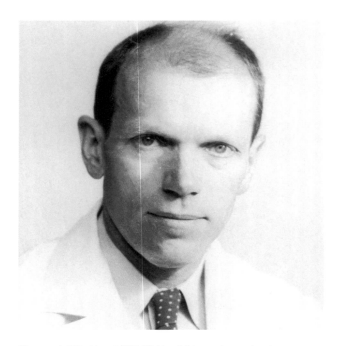

Figure 1.17 Harold Wolff. He did have the technology to run Darwin's experiment. He borrowed the G-machine at the US Army Air Corps laboratory in 1940. The headache did indeed disappear – as the patient lost consciousness. He is better known for his experiments with ergotamine tartrate (see Figure 1.18). Courtesy of the National Library of Medicine, Bethesda, USA

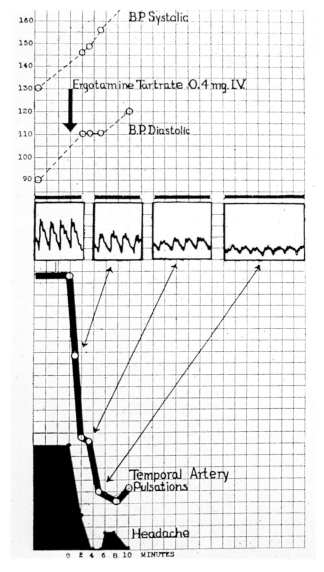

Figure 1.18 Illustration from Wolff's classic paper on the effect of ergotamine tartrate on pulsatility of cranial blood vessels and on migraine headache. Reproduced with permission from Graham JR, Wolff HG. Mechanisms of migraine headache and action of ergotamine tartrate. *Arch Neurol Psychiatr* 1938; 39:737–63

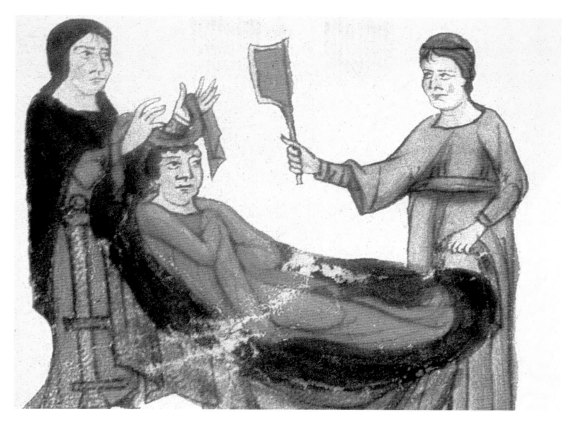

Figure 1.19 Mural from wall of Roman villa, circa 300 AD. The master of the house has migraine. One hand-maiden is applying a poultice of honey and opium (did they know back then that there are opioid receptors on peripheral nerves?), and another is fanning the master's brow

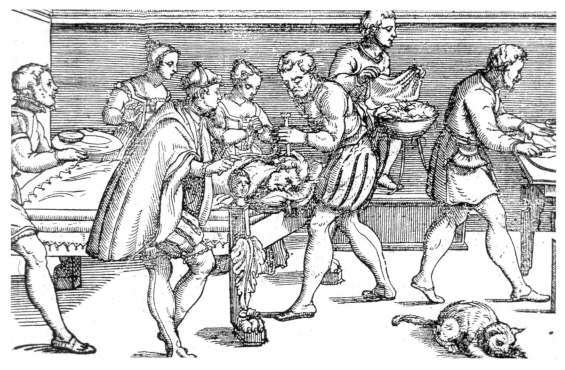

Figure 1.20 Illustration from Italian medieval manuscript, by Della Croce, dated 1583. The legend indicates that this man was trepanned for hemicrania. Outcome unknown. Note the cat in the lower right hand corner, that has caught a rat (the beginning of the aseptic method in the operating room?)

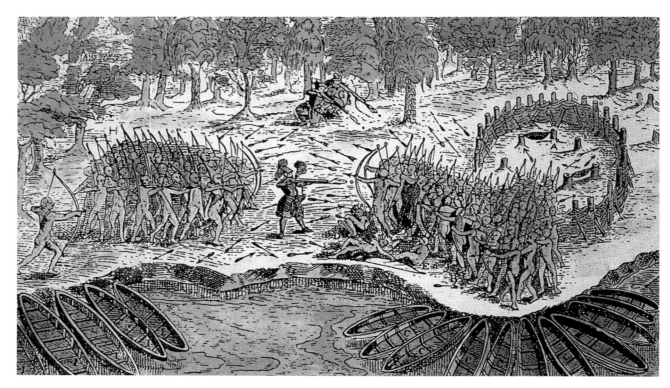

Figure 1.21 On July 30, 1609, Samuel de Champlain, a French explorer of New France (North America), was taken along by his Huron Indian hosts on a raid against the Mohawks, who lived on the shores of a large lake (Lake Champlain) in what is now upper New York State. There is a drawing by Champlain himself of the battle, in which he and his fellow Frenchmen won the day with their muskets. Towards the end of the battle, Champlain developed a severe migraine. See Figure 1.22

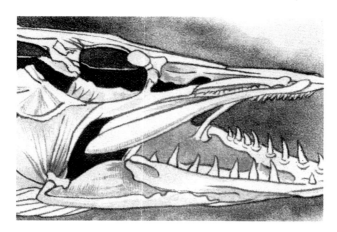

Figure 1.22 The victorious Hurons caught a gar pike in the lake, stripped its head of the flesh and instructed Champlain to rake his painful head with the sharp teeth, sufficient to draw blood. He did so, and his headache disappeared. Champlain took the head back to France with him, and gave it to the King of France, who also had migraine. We do not know if he ever used it

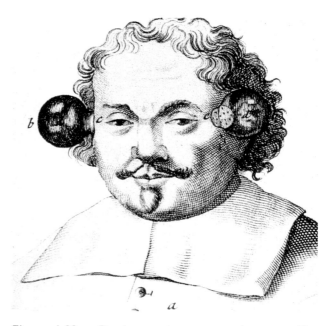

Figure 1.23 Dutch engraving, seventeenth century. The migraine sufferer has had puncture wounds put into his sore temples. Then heated glass globes are placed with their open mouths over the puncture wounds. As the globes cooled, a vacuum was set up, sucking the blood from the temples into the globes and relieving the headache. In this way, several patients could be treated at once (the first migraine clinic?)

WOLCOTT'S INSTANT PAIN ANNIHILATOR.

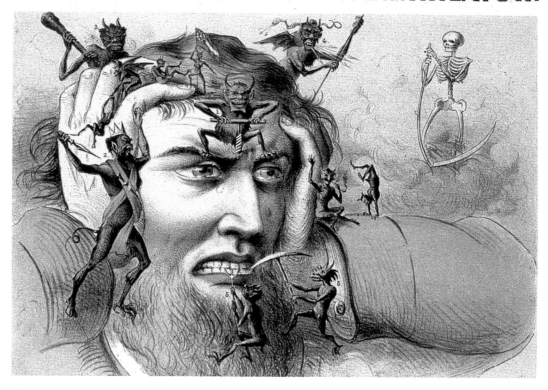

Figure 1.24 Advertisement from USA popular magazine (Harper's), 1863. Wolcott's Instant Pain Annihilator. Headache before Wolcott's

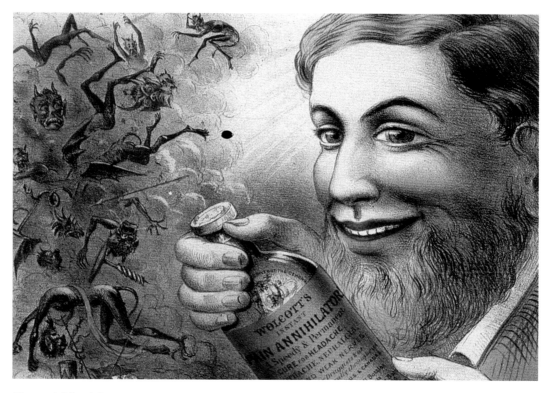

Figure 1.25 Advertisement continued. Headache gone (possible 2 h pain relief?) after Wolcott's

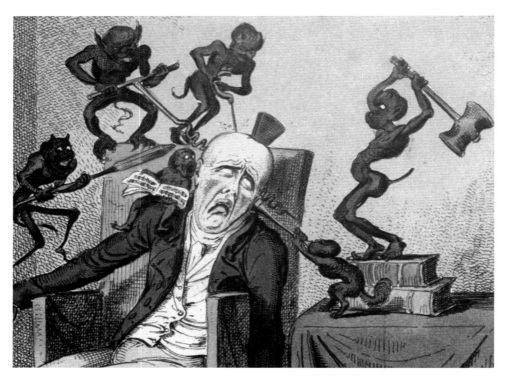

Figure 1.26 'Headache'. The colored etching by George Cruikshank (English, 1792–1878) after a design by Maryatt (London, 1819) dramatizes the impact of a headache of such intensity that one might almost venture to diagnose it as migraine. Reproduced with kind permission of Corbis Images, London, UK

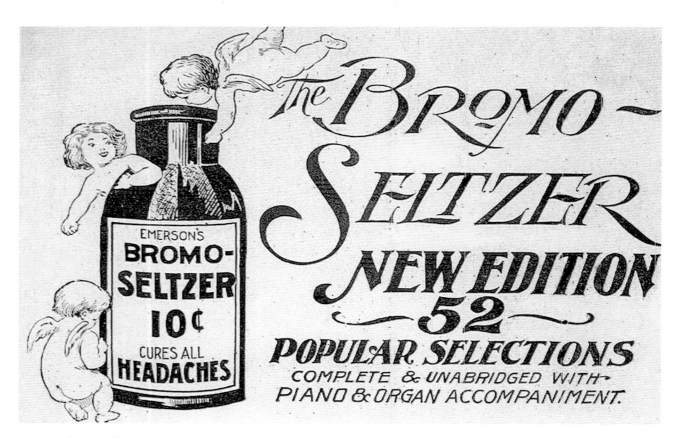

Figure 1.27 In 1888, Isaac E. Emerson, with his background in chemistry and pharmacy, conceived the idea of a headache remedy in his drugstore in Baltimore. The remedy was a granular effervescent salt he named 'Bromo-Seltzer'. Dispensing it to friends and customers at his drugstore, it soon became so successful that he abandoned his retail business to devote his time to the manufacture of his product. Eventually he established the Emerson Drug Company, incorporating it in Maryland in 1891

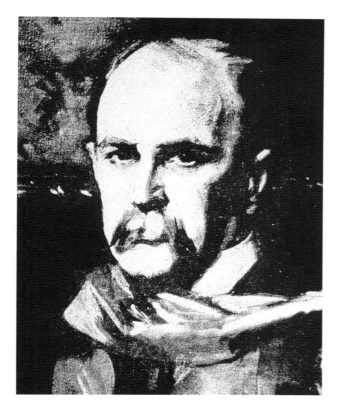

Figure 1.28 Sir William Osler, Professor of Medicine at Johns Hopkins University, who in his classic textbook (first edition 1892) opined that what we now call 'tension-type headache' was due to 'muscular rheumatism' of the scalp and neck. He called them 'indurative headaches'. The first to hypothesize the existence of 'muscle contraction headaches'

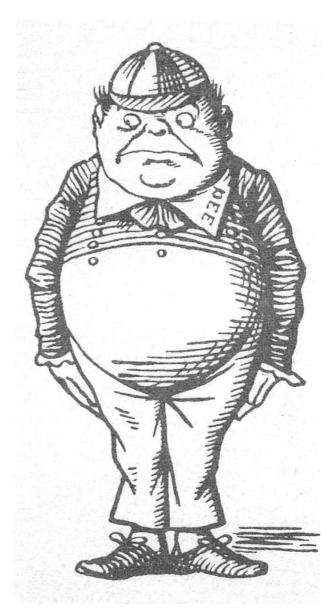

Figure 1.30 This is Tweedledee, famous for his statement: 'Generally I'm very brave, only today I happen to have a headache'! A John Tenniel illustration

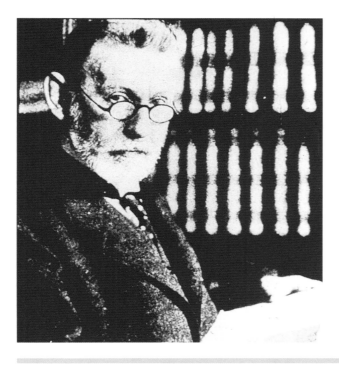

Figure 1.29 Paul Ehrlich, Nobel Prize winner in 1908, for work on immunology and receptors. Courtesy of the National Library of Medicine, Bethesda, USA

CLASSIFICATION OF HEADACHE DISORDERS, CRANIAL NEURALGIAS AND FACIAL PAIN

1. **Migraine**
   1.1 MIGRAINE WITHOUT AURA
   1.2 MIGRAINE WITH AURA
       Migraine with typical aura
       Migraine with prolonged aura
       Familial hemiplegic migraine
       Basilar migraine
       Migraine aura without headache
       Migraine with acute onset aura
   1.3 OPHTHALMOPLEGIC MIGRAINE
   1.4 RETINAL MIGRAINE
   1.5 CHILDHOOD PERIODIC SYNDROMES THAT MAY BE PRECURSORS TO OR ASSOCIATED WITH MIGRAINE
       Benign paroxysmal vertigo of childhood
       Alternating hemiplegia of childhood
   1.6 COMPLICATIONS OF MIGRAINE
       Status migrainosus
       Migrainous infarction
   1.7 MIGRAINOUS DISORDER NOT FULFILLING ABOVE CRITERIA

2. **Tension-type headache**
   2.1 EPISODIC TENSION-TYPE HEADACHE
       Episodic tension-type headache associated with disorder of pericranial muscles
       Episodic tension-type headache unassociated with disorder of pericranial muscles
   2.2 CHRONIC TENSION-TYPE HEADACHE
       Chronic tension-type headache associated with disorder of pericranial muscles
       Chronic tension-type headache unassociated with disorder of pericranial muscles
   2.3 HEADACHE OF THE TENSION-TYPE NOT FULFILLING ABOVE CRITERIA

3. **Cluster headache and chronic paroxysmal hemicrania**
   3.1 CLUSTER HEADACHE
       Cluster headache periodicity undetermined
       Episodic cluster headache
       Chronic cluster headache
           Unremitting from onset
           Evolved from episodic
   3.2 CHRONIC PAROXYSMAL HEMICRANIA
   3.3 CLUSTER HEADACHE-LIKE DISORDER NOT FULFILLING ABOVE CRITERIA

4. **Miscellaneous headaches unassociated with structural lesion**
   4.1 IDIOPATHIC STABBING HEADACHE
   4.2 EXTERNAL COMPRESSION HEADACHE
   4.3 COLD STIMULUS HEADACHE
       External application of a cold stimulus
       Ingestion of a cold stimulus
   4.4 BENIGN COUGH HEADACHE
   4.5 BENIGN EXERTIONAL HEADACHE
   4.6 HEADACHES ASSOCIATED WITH SEXUAL ACTIVITY
       Dull type
       Explosive type
       Postural type

5. **Headache associated with head trauma**
   5.1 ACUTE POST-TRAUMATIC HEADACHE
       With significant head trauma and/or confirmatory signs
       With minor head trauma and no confirmatory signs
   5.2 CHRONIC POST-TRAUMATIC HEADACHE
       With significant head trauma and/or confirmatory signs
       With minor head trauma and no confirmatory signs

6. **Headache associated with vascular disorders**
   6.1 ACUTE ISCHEMIC CEREBROVASCULAR DISEASE
       Transient ischemic attack (TIA)
       Thromboembolic stroke
   6.2 INTRACRANIAL HEMATOMA
       Intracerebral hematoma
       Subdural hematoma
       Epidural hematoma
   6.3 SUBARACHNOID HEMORRHAGE
   6.4 UNRUPTURED VASCULAR MALFORMATION
       Arteriovenous malformation
       Saccular aneurysm
   6.5 ARTERITIS
       Giant-cell arteritis
       Other systemic arteritides
       Primary intracranial arteritis
   6.6 CAROTID OR VERTEBRAL ARTERY PAIN
       Carotid or vertebral dissection
       Carotidynia (idiopathic)
       Post-endarterectomy headache
   6.7 VENOUS THROMBOSIS
   6.8 ARTERIAL HYPERTENSION
       Acute pressor response to exogenous agent
       Pheochromocytoma
       Malignant (accelerated) hypertension
       Pre-eclampsia and eclampsia
   6.9 HEADACHE ASSOCIATED WITH OTHER VASCULAR DISORDER

7. **Headache associated with non-vascular intracranial disorder**
   7.1 HIGH CEREBROSPINAL FLUID PRESSURE
       Benign intracranial hypertension
       High pressure hydrocephalus
   7.2 LOW CEREBROSPINAL FLUID PRESSURE
       Post-lumbar puncture headache
       Cerebrospinal fluid fistula headache
   7.3 INTRACRANIAL INFECTION
   7.4 INTRACRANIAL SARCOIDOSIS AND OTHER NON-INFECTIOUS INFLAMMATORY DISEASES

Figure 2.1   Classification of headache disorders, cranial neuralgias and facial pain published by the International Headache Society. Purple, primary headache disorders; blue, secondary headache disorders. Reproduced with permission from Headache

7.5 HEADACHE RELATED TO INTRATHECAL INJECTIONS
   Direct effect
   Due to chemical meningitis
7.6 INTRACRANIAL NEOPLASM
7.7 HEADACHE ASSOCIATED WITH OTHER INTRACRANIAL DISORDER

8. **Headache associated with substances or their withdrawal**
   8.1 HEADACHE INDUCED BY ACUTE SUBSTANCE USE OR EXPOSURE
      Nitrate/nitrite-induced headache
      Monosodium glutamate-induced headache
      Carbon monoxide-induced headache
      Alcohol-induced headache
      Other substances
   8.2 HEADACHE INDUCED BY CHRONIC SUBSTANCE USE OR EXPOSURE
      Ergotamine-induced headache
      Analgesics abuse headache
      Other substances
   8.3 HEADACHE FROM SUBSTANCE WITHDRAWAL (ACUTE USE)
      Alcohol withdrawal headache (hangover)
      Other substances
   8.4 HEADACHE FROM SUBSTANCE WITHDRAWAL (CHRONIC USE)
      Ergotamine withdrawal headache
      Caffeine withdrawal headache
      Narcotics abstinence headache
      Other substances
   8.5 HEADACHE ASSOCIATED WITH SUBSTANCES BUT WITH UNCERTAIN MECHANISM
      Birth control pills or estrogens
      Other substances

9. **Headache associated with non-cephalic infection**
   9.1 VIRAL INFECTION
      Focal non-cephalic
      Systemic
   9.2 BACTERIAL INFECTION
      Focal non-cephalic
      Systemic (septicemia)
   9.3 HEADACHE RELATED TO OTHER INFECTION

10. **Headache associated with metabolic disorder**
   10.1 HYPOXIA
      High altitude headache
      Hypoxic headache (low pressure environment, pulmonary disease causing hypoxia)
      Sleep apnea headache
   10.2 HYPERCAPNIA
   10.3 MIXED HYPOXIA AND HYPERCAPNIA
   10.4 HYPOGLYCEMIA
   10.5 DIALYSIS
   10.6 HEADACHE RELATED TO OTHER METABOLIC ABNORMALITY

11. **Headache or facial pain associated with disorder of cranium, neck, eyes, ears, nose, sinuses, teeth, mouth or other facial or cranial structures**
   11.1 CRANIAL BONE
   11.2 NECK
      Cervical spine
      Retropharyngeal tendinitis
   11.3 EYES
      Acute glaucoma
      Refractive errors
      Heterophoria or heterotropia
   11.4 EARS
   11.5 NOSE AND SINUSES
      Acute sinus headache
      Other diseases of nose or sinuses
   11.6 TEETH, JAWS AND RELATED STRUCTURES
   11.7 TEMPOROMANDIBULAR JOINT DISEASE (FUNCTIONAL DISORDERS ARE CODED TO GROUP 2)

12. **Cranial neuralgias, nerve trunk pain and deafferentation pain**
   12.1 PERSISTENT (IN CONTRAST TO TIC-LIKE) PAIN OF CRANIAL NERVE ORIGIN
      Compression or distortion of cranial nerves and second or third cervical roots
      Demyelination of cranial nerves
         Optic neuritis (retro-bulbar neuritis)
      Infarction of cranial nerves
         Diabetic neuritis
      Inflammation of cranial nerves
         Herpes zoster
         Chronic post-herpetic neuralgia
      Tolosa-Hunt syndrome
      Neck-tongue syndrome
      Other causes of persistent pain of cranial nerve origin
   12.2 TRIGEMINAL NEURALGIA
      Idiopathic trigeminal neuralgia
      Symptomatic trigeminal neuralgia
         Compression of trigeminal root or ganglion
         Central lesions
   12.3 GLOSSOPHARYNGEAL NEURALGIA
      Idiopathic glossopharyngeal neuralgia
      Symptomatic glossopharyngeal neuralgia
   12.4 NERVUS INTERMEDIUS NEURALGIA
   12.5 SUPERIOR LARYNGEAL NEURALGIA
   12.6 OCCIPITAL NEURALGIA
   12.7 CENTRAL CAUSES OF HEAD AND FACIAL PAIN OTHER THAN TIC DOULOUREUX
      Anesthesia dolorosa
      Thalamic pain
   12.8 Facial pain not fulfilling criteria in groups 11 and 12

13. **Headache not classifiable**

Figure 2.1 *Continued* Classification Committee of the International Headache Society. Classification and diagnostic criteria for headache disorders, cranial neuralgias and facial pain. *Cephalalgia* 1988;8(Suppl 7):1–96

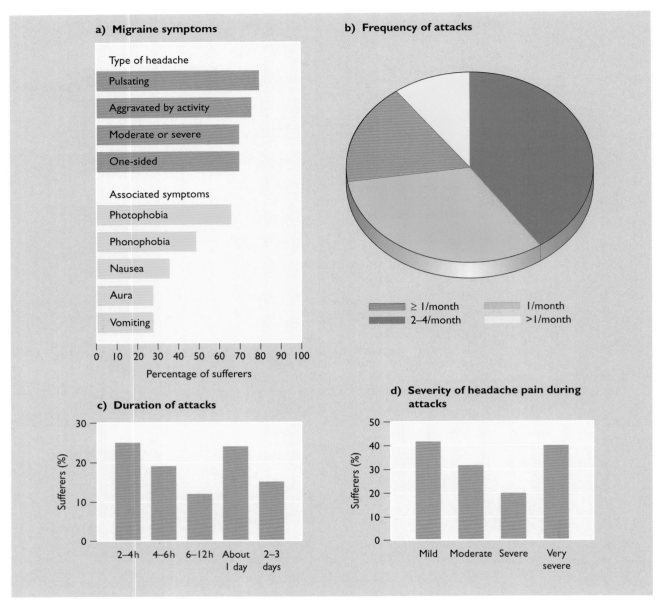

Figure 3.1 Migraine characteristics from population studies of migraine epidemiology using the diagnostic criteria of the International Headache Society (IHS). (a) Adapted with permission from Micieli G. Suffering in silence. In: Edmeads J, ed. *Migraine: A Brighter Future*, 1993:1–7, with permission of Cambridge Medical Publications; (b) to (d) data derived from Henry P, Michel P, Brochet B, *et al.* A nationwide survey of migraine in France: prevalence and clinical features in adults. *Cephalalgia* 1992;12:229–37

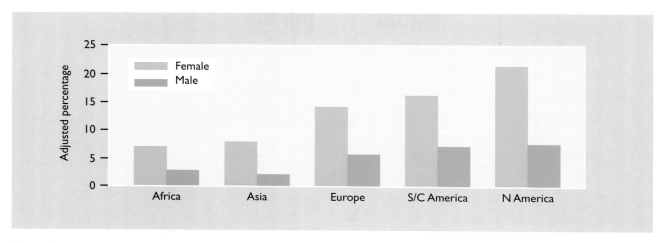

Figure 3.2 Adjusted prevalence of migraine by geographic area. Adapted with permission from Stewart WF, Lipton RB, Celentano DD, Reed ML. Prevalence of migraine headache in the United States. Relation to age, income, race, and other sociodemographic factors. *JAMA* 1992;267:64–9

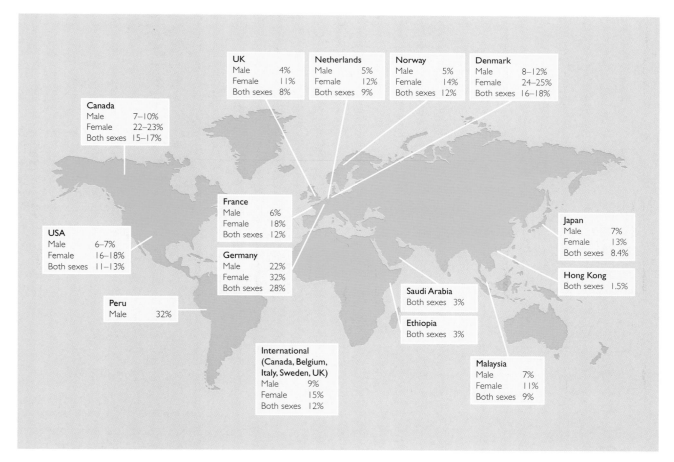

Figure 3.3 Estimates of migraine prevalence in studies using the diagnostic criteria of the International Headache Society (IHS). Adapted with kind permission of Richard B. Lipton

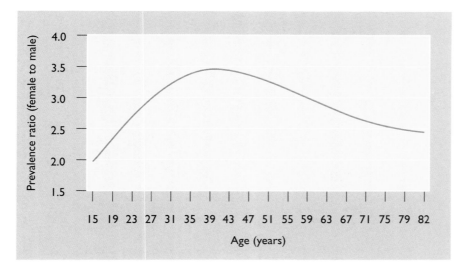

Figure 3.4 Women are more commonly affected by headache than men. This graph shows the prevalence ratio of migraine headache (females to males) over a lifetime. Adapted with permission from Lipton RB, Stewart WF. Migraine in the United States: a review of epidemiology and health care use. *Neurology* 1993;43(Suppl 3):S6–10

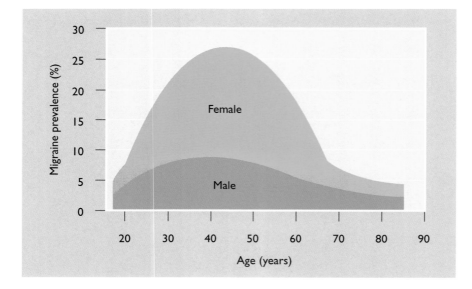

Figure 3.5 Age-specific prevalence of migraine among women and men in a US study. Adapted with permission from Stewart WF, Lipton RB, Celentano DD, Reed ML. Prevalence of migraine headache in the United States. *JAMA* 1992;267:64–9

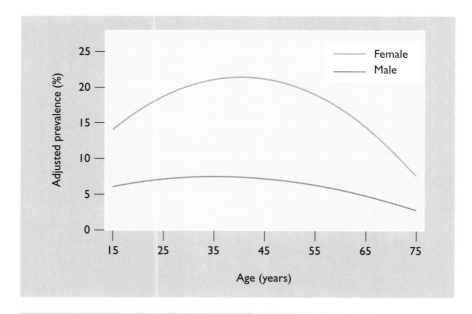

Figure 3.6 Age- and sex-specific prevalence of migraine based on a meta-analytic summary of 18 population-based studies. Adapted with permission from Scher AI, Stewart WF, Lipton RB. Migraine and headache: A meta-analytic approach. In: Crombie I, ed. *Epidemiology of Pain*. Seattle: IASP Press, 1999:159–70

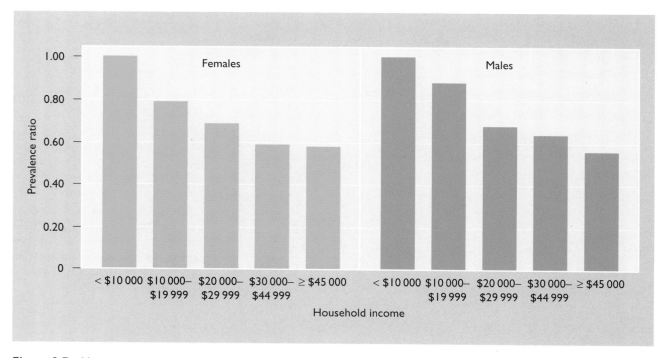

Figure 3.7 Migraine prevalence is inversely proportional to income, with the low income groups having the highest prevalence. Adapted with permission from Lipton RB, Stewart WF, Celentano DD, Reed ML. Undiagnosed migraine headaches. A comparison of symptom-based and reported physician diagnosis. *Arch Intern Med* 1992;152:1273–8

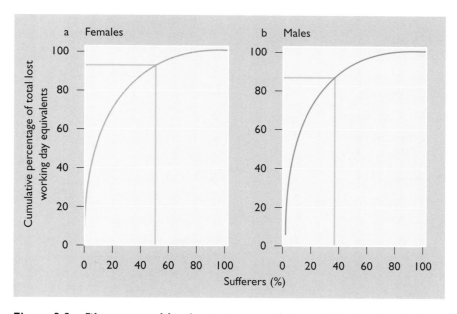

Figure 3.8 Fifty percent of female migraineurs and almost 40% of male migraineurs accounted for approximately 90% of lost working day equivalents. Adapted with permission from Stewart WF, Lipton RB, Simon D. Work-related disability: Results from the American Migraine Study. *Cephalalgia* 1996;16:231–8

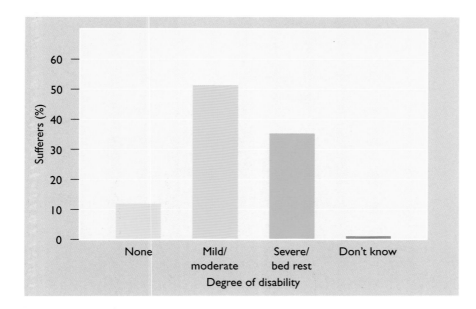

Figure 3.9 Degree of disability due to migraine in a US study. Adapted with permission from Stewart WF, Lipton RB, Celentano DD, Reed ML. Prevalence of migraine headache in the United States. *JAMA* 1992;267:64–9

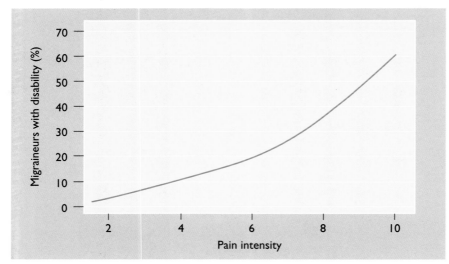

Figure 3.10 Relationship between disability and headache pain intensity in a group of migraine sufferers. Adapted with permission from Stewart WF, Shechter A, Lipton RB. Migraine heterogeneity. Disability, pain intensity and attack frequency and duration. *Neurology* 1994;44:24–39

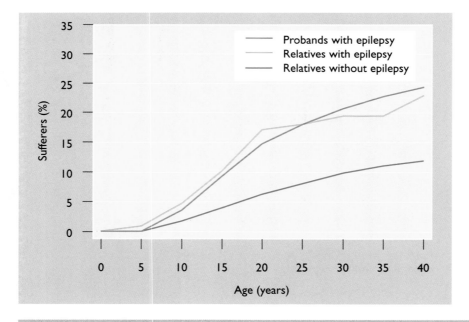

Figure 3.11 Cumulative incidence of migraine headache, by age, in probands with epilepsy (red), relatives with epilepsy (yellow) and relatives without epilepsy (green). Adapted with permission from Ottman R, Lipton RB. Comorbidity of migraine and epilepsy. *Neurology* 1994;44:2105–10

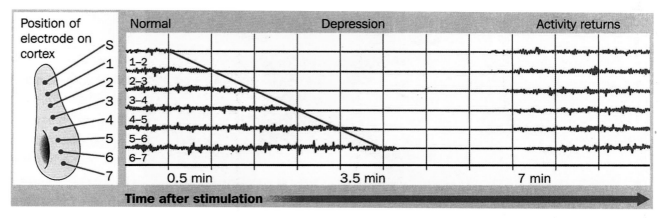

Figure 4.1 Leao found that noxious stimulation of the exposed cortex of a rabbit produced a spreading decrease in electrical activity that moved at a rate of 2–3 mm/min. Reading from the rabbit cortex illustrating spreading depression of EEG activity. Reproduced with permission from Leao AAP. Spreading depression of activity in cerebral cortex. *J Neurophysiol* 1944;7:359–90

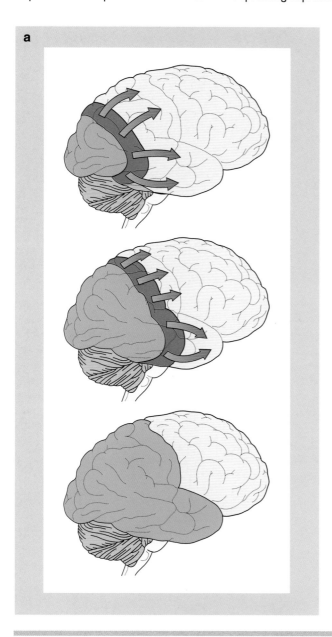

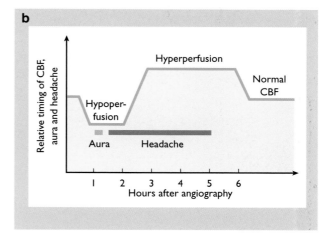

Figure 4.2 Line drawing (panel a) of the spreading oligemia observed with studies of cerebral blood flow (CBF) during aura after Lauritzen. Adapted with permission from Lauritzen M. Cortical spreading depression as a putative migraine mechanism. *Trends Neurosci* 1987;10:8–13, with permission from Elsevier Science. Panel b illustrates the variable time course and relationship of the changes in cerebral blood flow and the symptomatology of migraine. Adapted with permission from Olesen J, Friberg L, Skyhoj-Olesen T, *et al.* Timing and topography of cerebral blood flow, aura and headache during migraine attacks. *Ann Neurol* 1990;28:791–8

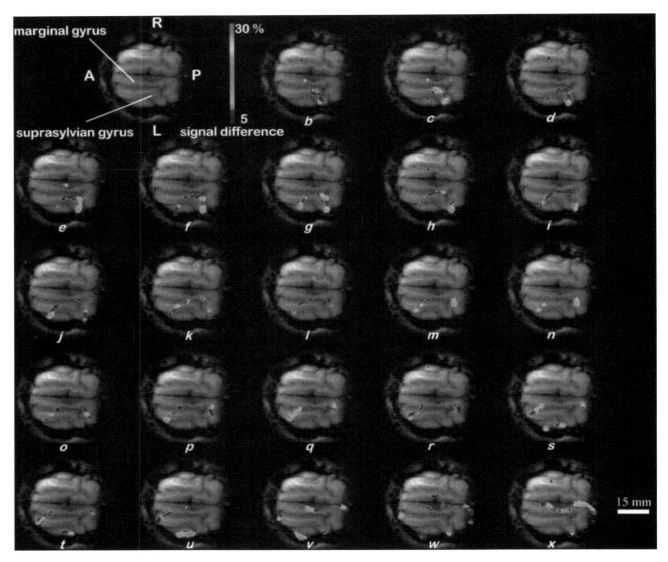

Figure 4.3 Propagation of cortical spreading depression (CSD) across the surface of the cat brain *in vivo*. Top left, control, horizontal, gradient-echo anatomic image depicting the suprasylvian and marginal gyri. Remaining images (b–x): coloured overlays, shown at 10 s intervals starting about 50 s after KCl application, represent elliptical regions of reduced diffusion travelling away from the KCl application site with a velocity of 3.2 ± 0.1 mm/min (mean ± SEM of 5 measurements). Over the first eleven frames (b–l) the wave travels both rostrally and caudally along the suprasylvian gyrus; when it reaches the caudal junction of the two gyri (m–s), it appears to pass into the marginal gyrus (t–x); likewise, rostrally, the wave passes first (r–x) into the ectosylvian gyrus where it dissipates (v–x) and then into the marginal gyrus (t–x). Waves were never detected in the contralateral hemisphere. A, anterior; P, posterior; R, right; L, left; overlays were obtained by subtracting a baseline image from the high-b images obtained in the DWEP sequence and transforming the signal difference into a percentage change (blue 5%, red 30%). Scale bar, 15 mm. This image represents the first reported detection of CSD with magnetic resonance imaging (MRI) in a species which shares with man a complex, gyrencephalic brain structure. Reproduced with permission from James MF, Smith MI, Bockhorst KH, *et al*. Cortical spreading depression in the gyrencephalic feline brain studied by magnetic resonance imaging. *J Physiol* 1999;519:415–25

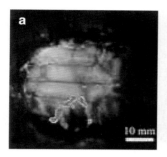
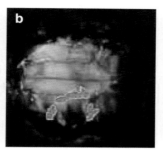
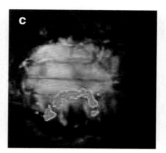
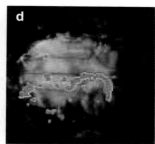

Figure 4.4 Spreading depression: A model of migraine. Colored overlays of changes in blood oxygenation in an experimental model of cortical spreading depression. Overlays a–d represent the points 0.5, 1.0, 1.4 and 5.1 min post-induction. Reproduced with permission from James MF, Smith MI, Bockhorst KH, et al. Cortical spreading depression in the gyrencephalic feline brain studied by magnetic resonance imaging. *J Physiol* 1999;519:415–25

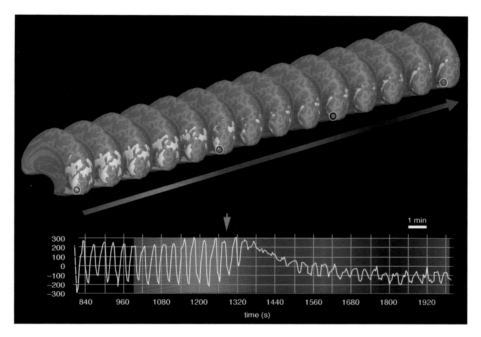

Figure 4.5 Blood oxygenation level-dependent (BOLD) changes during an exercise-triggered migraine visual aura. Time-dependent BOLD activity changes from a single region of interest in the primary visual cortex (VI), aquired before and during episodes of induced visual aura. The upper panel shows a series of anatomic images, including BOLD activity on 'inflated' cortical hemispheres showing the medial bank (similar to a conventional mid-sagittal view). Images were sampled at 32 s intervals, showing the same region of interest (circle) in VI. The lower panel shows the MR signal perturbation over time from the circled region of interest. Variations in time are color-coded (deep red to magenta) and the four-colored circles match corresponding times within the VI region of interest. Prior to the onset of the aura, the BOLD response to visual stimulation shows a normal, oscillating activation pattern. Following the onset of aura (red arrow), the BOLD response shows a marked increase in mean level and a marked suppression to light modulation followed by a partial recovery of the response to light modulation at a decreased mean level. Reproduced with kind permission of Margarita Sanchez del Rio

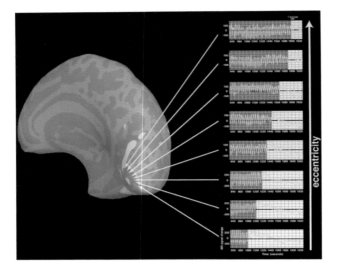

Figure 4.6 Spreading suppression of cortical activation during migraine visual aura. Data from the same patient as in Figure 4.5. The posterior medial aspect of the occipital lobe is shown in an 'inflated cortex' format. The cortical sulci and gyri appear in darker and lighter gray respectively, on a computationally inflated surface. MR signal changes over time are shown on the right. Each time course was recorded from one in a sequence of voxels which were sampled along the calcarine sulcus in V1, from the posterior pole to the more anterior location, as indicated by the arrow. A similar BOLD response was found within all the extrastriate areas, differing only in the time of onset of the MR perturbation. The MR perturbations developed earlier in the foveal representation, compared to the more eccentric representation of the retinotropic visual cortex. This was consistent with the progression of the aura from central to peripheral eccentricities in the corresponding visual field. Reproduced with kind permission of Margarita Sanchez del Rio

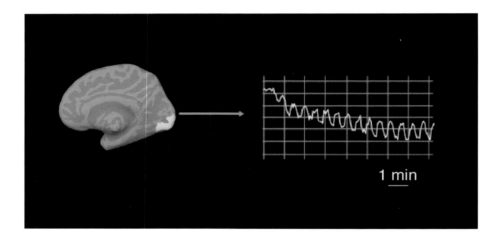

Figure 4.7 BOLD changes during spontaneous migraine visual aura. Data from a spontaneous attack captured approximately 18 min after the onset of the visual symptoms affecting the right hemifield. The data represent the time course in the left visual area V1, at an eccentricity of approximately 20° of visual angle. BOLD signal changes resemble the changes observed at a similar time point in Figure 4.5. Reproduced with kind permission of Margarita Sanchez del Rio

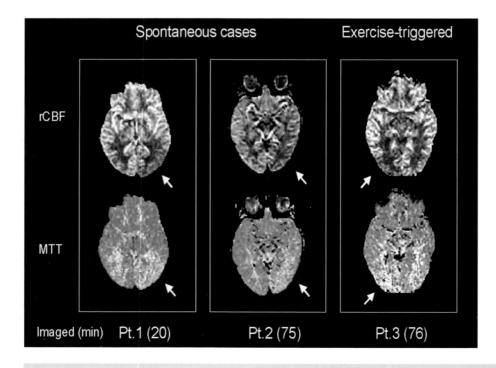

Figure 4.8 Perfusion weighted imaging (PWI) during migraine with aura attacks. PWI maps obtained at different time points during migraine with aura attacks during the presence of the stereotypical visual aura (patient 1, approximately 20 min after onset of visual symptoms) and after resolution of the aura and into the headache phase (patients 2 and 3). In all cases a perfusion defect (decreased rCBF and rCBV, the latter not shown, and increased MTT) was observed in the occipital cortex contralateral to the visual field defect. rCBF, reduced cerebral blood flow; rCBV, regional cerebral blood volume; MTT, mean transit time. Reproduced with kind permission of Margarita Sanchez del Rio

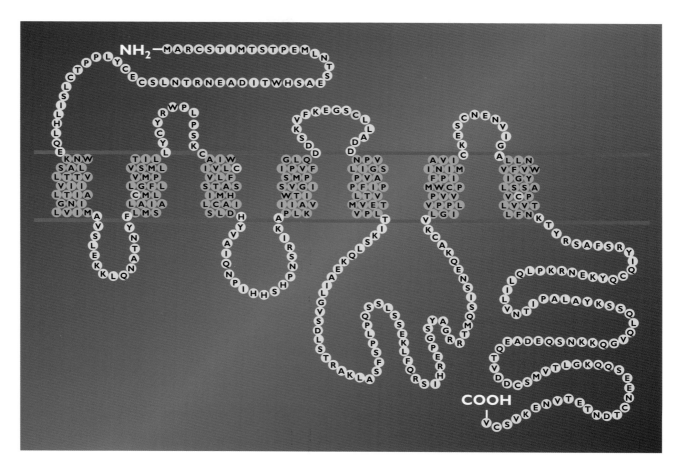

Figure 4.9 Schematic representation of the primary sequence of the 5-HT$_2$ receptor. Reproduced from Hartig PR. Molecular biology of 5-HT receptor. *Trends Pharmacol Sci* 1989;10:64–9, with permission from Elsevier Science

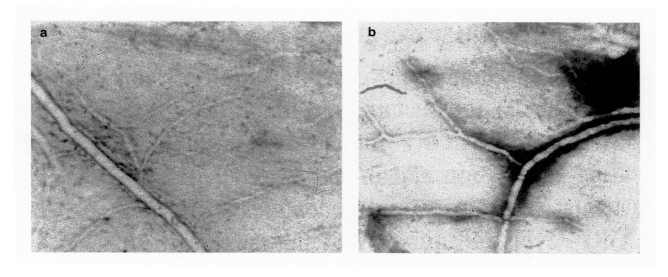

Figure 4.10 Trigeminal stimulation in the rat produces plasma protein extravasation. 5-Hydroxytryptamine receptor agonists for the abortive treatment of vascular headaches block this effect. (a) control; (b) stimulated. Reproduced from Buzzi MG, Dimitriadou V, Theoharides TC, Moskowitz MA. 5-Hydroxytryptamine receptor agonists for the abortive treatment of vascular headaches block mast cell, endothelial and platelet activation within the rat dura mater after trigeminal stimulation. *Brain Res* 1992;583:137–49, with permission from Elsevier Science

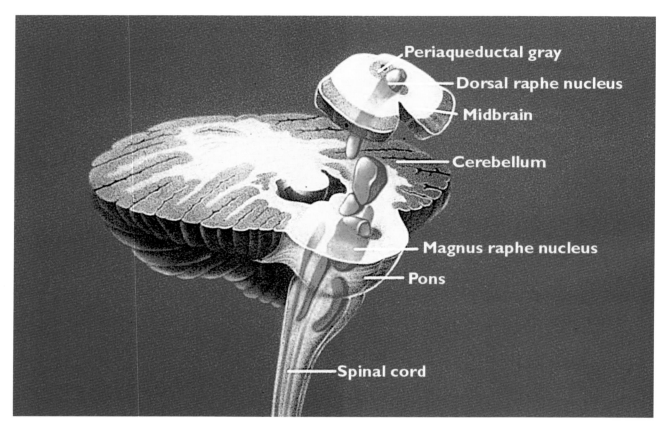

Figure 4.11 Brainstem nuclei thought to be involved in migraine generation include the periaqueductal gray matter and dorsal raphe nucleus

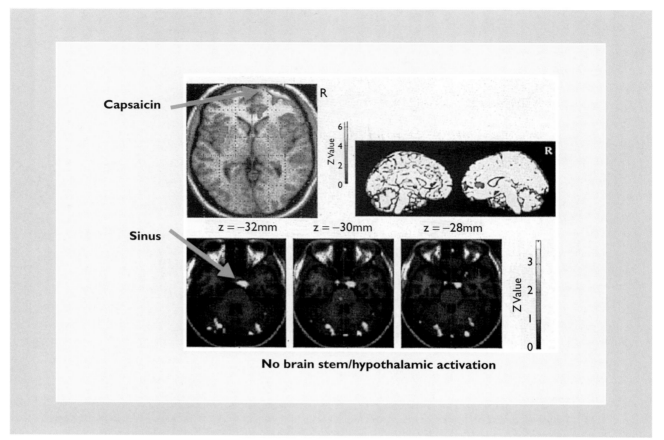

Figure 4.12 An experimental pain study was conducted in healthy volunteers to further test whether brain stem neuronal activation during migraine is specific to the generation of migraine symptoms. In this study, capsaicin was injected subcutaneously into the right forehead to evoke a painful burning sensation in the first division of the trigeminal nerve. The monoaminergic brain stem regions (raphe nucleus and the locus coeruleus) and the periaqueductal gray were not activated in the acute pain state compared to the pain-free state. Thus, brain stem activation during a migraine attack is probably not a generalized response to head pain but instead represents sites in the nervous system that may give rise to migraine symptomatology. Adapted with permission from May A, Kaube H, Buchel C, *et al*. Experimental cranial pain elicited by capsaicin: a PET study. *Pain* 1998;74:61–6

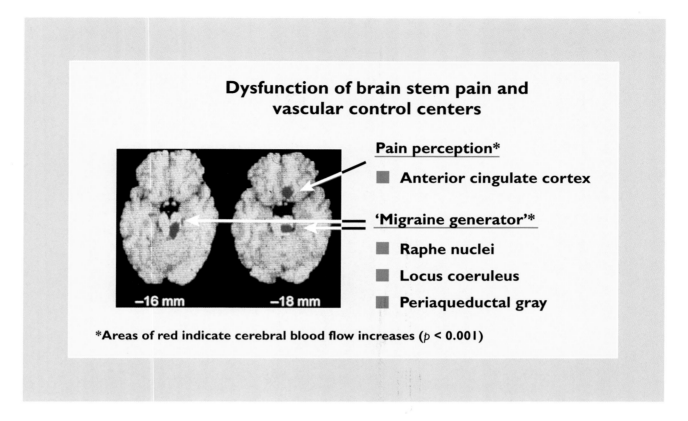

Figure 4.13 The development of migraine, e.g. episodes in patients undergoing surgery to implant electrodes in the periaqueductal gray and raphe nuclei for the treatment of chronic pain, generated the hypothesis that CNS dysfunction early in the migraine attack could provoke changes in these brain stem nuclei. Weiller *et al.* used positron emission tomography (PET) to examine the changes in regional cerebral blood flow, an index of neuronal activity, during spontaneous migraine attacks. The left panel above is a PET scan from an individual during a migraine attack treated acutely with sumatriptan. The scan depicts neuronal activity in a section through the brain stem. The authors of this study reported that monoaminergic brain stem regions (raphe nucleus comprising serotonergic neurons and the locus coeruleus comprising noradrenergic neurons) and the periaqueductal gray are selectively activated during a migraine attack. When this patient used subcutaneous sumatriptan to acutely relieve his headache pain, the brain stem centers continued to appear active on the follow-up PET scans. By contrast, the anterior cingulate cortex, a region thought to be involved in processing affective components of pain, was also activated during spontaneous migraine attacks, and this activation was reduced concomitantly with headache pain relief after administration of sumatriptan. Taken together, these observations suggest that the raphe nucleus, locus coeruleus and the periaqueductal gray are regions that may be involved in the generation of headache pain and associated symptoms during a migraine attack. Adapted with permission from Weiller C, May A, Limmroth V, *et al.* Brain stem activation in spontaneous human migraine attacks. *Nat Med* 1995;1:658–60

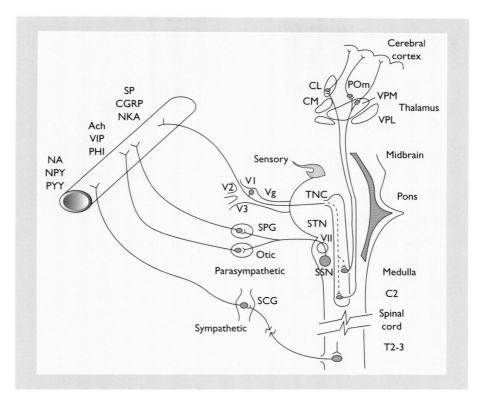

Figure 4.14 Brainstem nuclei and their transmitters. Ach, acetylcholine; C2, second cervical segment of the spinal cord; CGRP, calcitonin gene-related peptide; CL, centrolateral nucleus of thalamus; CM, centromedial nucleus of thalamus; NA, noradrenaline; NKA, neurokinin A; NPY, neuropeptide Y; Otic, otic ganglion; PHI, peptide histidine isoleucine (methionine in man); POm, medial nucleus of the posterior complex; PYY, peptide YY; SCG, superior cervical ganglion; SP, substance P; SPG, sphenopalatine ganglion; SSN, superior salivatory nucleus; STN, spinal trigeminal nucleus; T2-3, second and third thoracic segments of the spinal cord; TNC, trigeminal nucleus caudalis; VII, seventh cranial nerve (parasympathetic outflow); VIP, vasoactive intestinal polypeptide; VPL, ventroposterolateral nucleus of thalamus; VPM, ventroposteromedial nucleus of thalamus; Vg, trigeminal ganglion; VI-3, first, second and third divisions of the trigeminal nerve. Reproduced with permission from Goadsby PJ, Zagami AS, Lambert GA. Neural processing of craniovascular pain: a synthesis of the central structures involved in migraine. *Headache* 1991;31:365–71

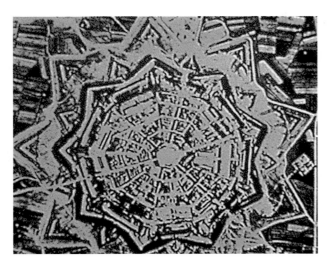

Figure 5.1 Fortification spectra seen in migraine visual auras have been compared to the aerial view of the fortified, walled city of Palmanova, Italy. Reproduced with permission from Silberstein SD, Lipton RB, Goadsby PJ. *Headache in Clinical Practice*. Oxford, UK: Isis Medical Media, 1998:64

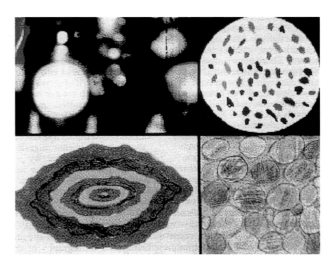

Figure 5.2 Migraine visual auras are very similar to epileptic visual hallucinations seen here. Reproduced from Panayiotopoulos CP. Elementary visual hallucinations in migraine and epilepsy. *J Neurol Neurosurg Psychiatr* 1994;57: 1371–4, with permission from the BMJ Publishing Group

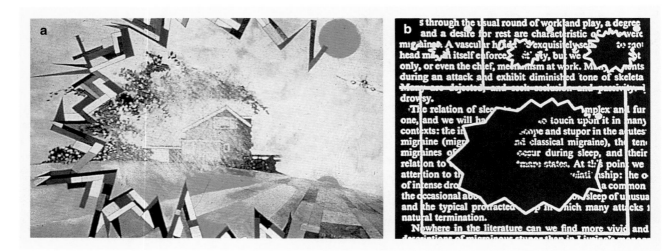

Figure 5.3 (a) An artist's representation of his visual disturbance during a migraine attack. In this the fortification spectrum is part of a formal design but still maintains a crescentic shape. There is also an associated partial visual loss. (b) An artist's representation similar to one of the images in Sir William Gowers' 1904 paper showing a progressive central scotoma with a jagged edge. The scotoma gradually increases to fill most of the central field. Reproduced with permission from Wilkinson M, Robinson D. Migraine art. *Cephalalgia* 1985;5:151–7

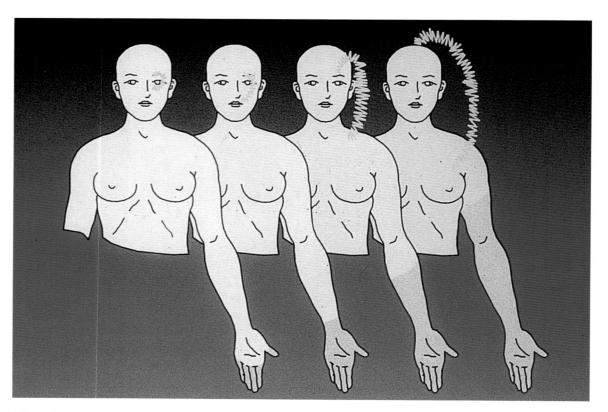

Figure 5.4 Paresthesias are the second most common migraine aura. Adapted from Spierings ELH. Symptomatology and pathogenesis. In: *Management of Migraine*. Boston, MA: Butterworth-Heinemann, 1996:7–19

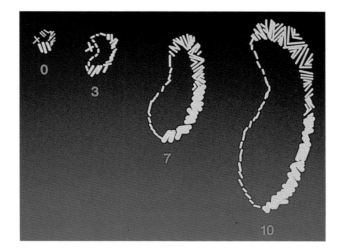

Figure 5.5 Fortification spectra as depicted by Lashley. An arch of scintillating lights, usually but not always beginning near the point of fixation, may form into a herring bone-like pattern that expands to encompass an increasing portion of the visual hemifield. It migrates across the visual field with a scintillating edge of often zigzag, flashing or occasionally colored phenomena. Reproduced with permission from Lashley K. Patterns of cerebral integration indicated by the scotomas of migraine. *Arch Neurol Psychiatr* 1941;46:331–9

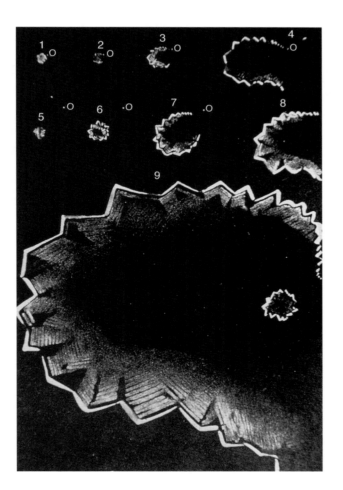

Figure 5.6 Migraine aura. 1–4, Early stages of sinistral teichopsia beginning close to the sight point, as seen in the dark. The letter O marks the sight point in every figure; 5–8, a similar series of the early stages of sinistral teichopsia beginning a few degrees below and to the left of the sight point; 9, sinistral teichopsia fully developed. Beginning of a secondary attack, which never attains full development, until it arises on the opposite side

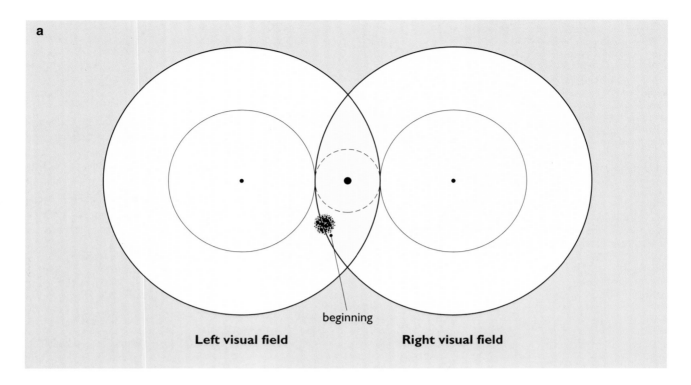

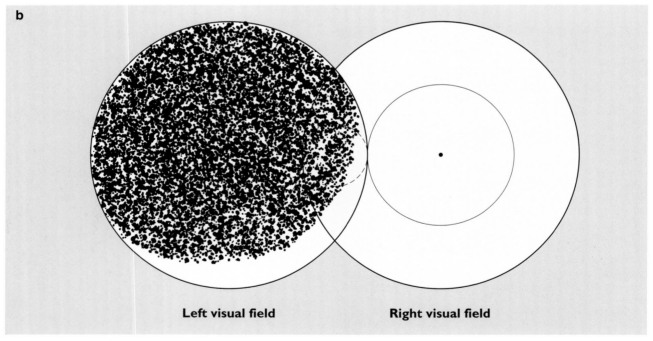

Figure 5.7 (a) and (b) Adapted from drawings by Professor Leao depicting an expanding hemianopsia as seen by a patient experiencing migraine visual aura, with kind permission of Luiz Paulo de Queiroz

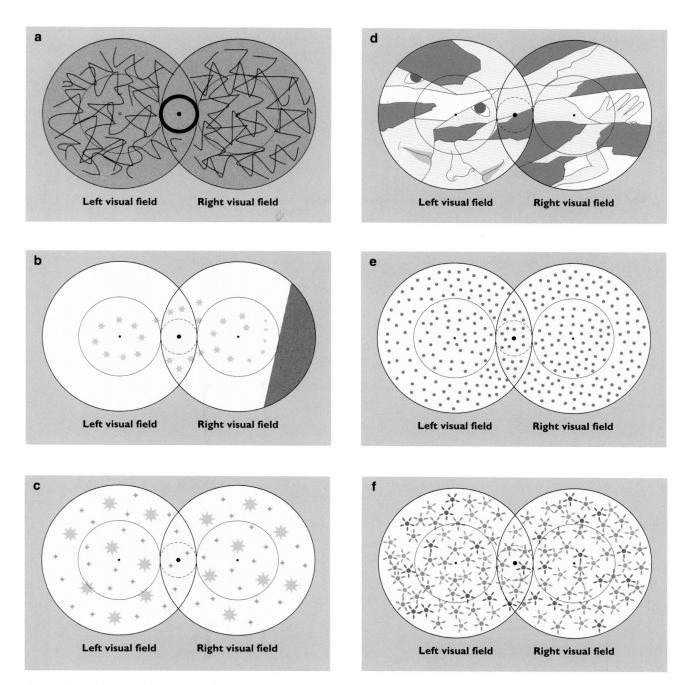

Figure 5.8 (a) to (f) Adapted from drawings by Professor Leao depicting a variety of visual auras described by patients, with kind permission of Luiz Paulo de Queiroz

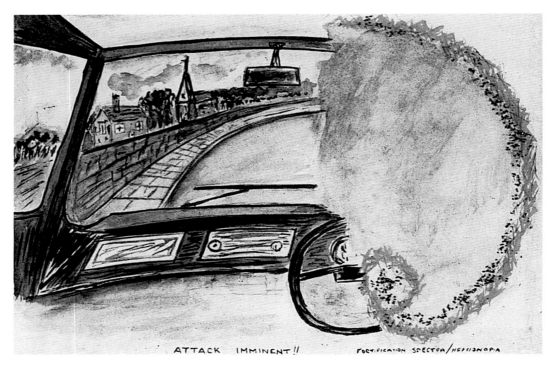

Figure 5.9 Motorist's right-sided hemianopic loss of vision, the scotomatous area being surrounded by a crescentic area of brighter lights. Reproduced with permission from Wilkinson M, Robinson D. Migraine art. *Cephalalgia* 1985;5:151–7

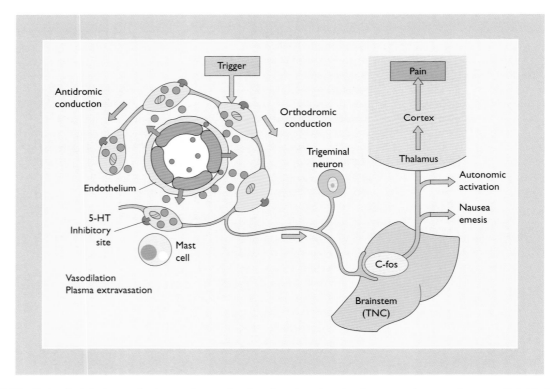

Figure 5.10 Pathophysiologic mechanism and postulated anti-nociceptive site for sumatriptan and ergot alkaloids in vascular headaches. The triggers for headache activate perivascular trigeminal axons, which release vasoactive neuropeptides to promote neurogenic inflammation (vasodilation, plasma extravasation, mast cell degranulation). Ortho- and antidromic conduction along trigeminovascular fibers spreads the inflammatory response to adjacent tissues and transmits nociceptive information towards the trigeminal nucleus caudalis and higher brain centers for the registration of pain. TNC, trigeminal nucleus caudalis. Adapted from Moskowitz MA. Neurogenic versus vascular mechanisms of sumatriptan and ergot alkaloids in migraine. *Trends Pharmacol Sci* 1992;13:307–11, with permission from Elsevier Science

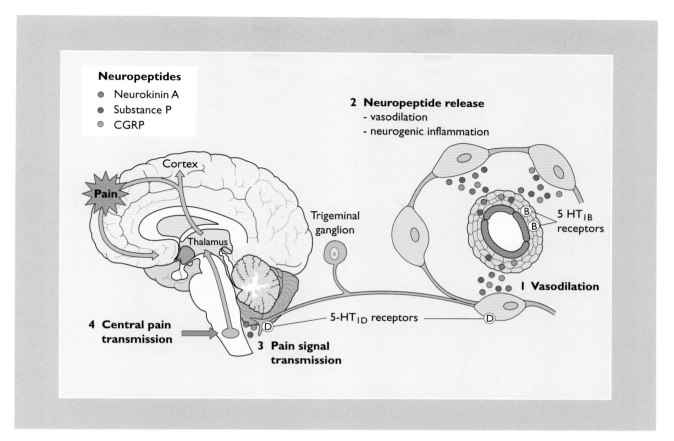

Figure 5.11 A primary dysfunction of brain stem pain and vascular control centers elicits a cascade of secondary changes in vascular regulation within pain-producing intracranial structures that ultimately manifests in headache pain and associated symptoms. A synthesis of these views and observations forms the neurovascular hypothesis of migraine. It is critical to understand the anatomy of the trigeminal vascular system and the pathophysiologic events that arise during a migraine attack before considering the proposed mechanisms of action of acute therapies. Current theories suggest that there are several key steps in the generation of migraine pain: (1) Intracranial meningeal blood vessel dilation which activates perivascular sensory trigeminal nerves. (2) Vasoactive neuropeptide release from activated trigeminal sensory nerves. These peptides can worsen and perpetuate any existing vasodilation, setting up a vicious cycle that increases sensory nerve activation and intensifies headache pain. The peptides include substance P (increased vascular permeability), neurokinin A (dilation and permeability changes) and calcitonin gene-related peptide (CGRP; long-lasting vasodilation). (3) Pain impulses from activated peripheral sensory nerves are relayed to second-order sensory neurons within the trigeminal nucleus caudalis in the brain stem and upper cervical spinal cord (C1 and C2, trigeminocervical complex). (4) Headache pain signals ascend to the thalamus, via the quintothalamic tract which decussates in the brain stem, and on to higher cortical centers where migraine pain is registered and perceived. Adapted with permission from Hargreaves RJ, Shepheard SL. Pathophysiology of migraine – new insights. *Can J Neurol Sci* 1999;26(Suppl 3):S12–19

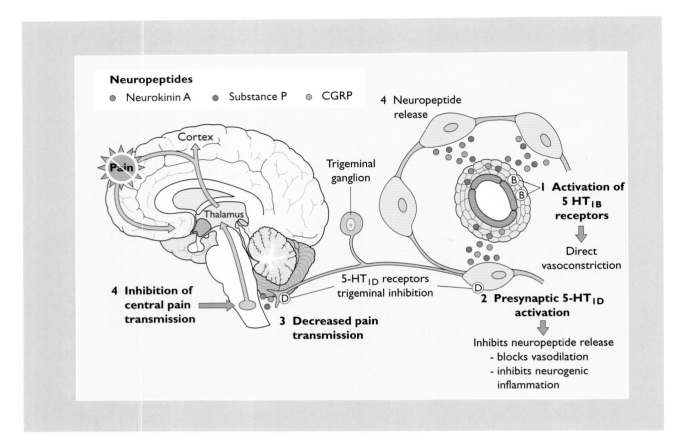

Figure 5.12 Increased knowledge of 5-HT receptor distribution within the trigeminovascular system has led to the introduction of highly effective serotonergic anti-migraine drug therapies. Detailed molecular biology mapping of mRNA (RT-PCR and *in situ* hybridization) and immunohistochemical studies of recepter proteins have revealed populations of vasoconstrictor 5-HT$_{1B}$ receptors on the smooth muscle of human meningeal blood vessels. Thus, agonists of 5-HT$_{1B}$ receptors, which cause vasoconstriction, are ideally placed to reverse the dilation of meningeal vessels that is thought to occur during a migraine attack (see 1). 5-HT$_{1B}$ receptors have also been found on human coronary arteries making it important to establish the relative contribution of this subtype to the contractile response in coronary arteries compared with the target meningeal blood vessels. While 5-HT$_{1F}$ mRNA has also been demonstrated in human blood vessels, there appears to be no expression of functional receptors since 5-HT$_{1F}$ agonists appear devoid of vasoconstrictor effects. Immunohistochemical mapping studies on the localization of 5-HT$_{1D}$ and 5-HT$_{1F}$ receptor proteins in human trigeminal nerves have shown that 5-HT$_{1D}$ and 5-HT$_{1F}$ receptors are present on trigeminal nerves projecting peripherally to the dural vasculature and centrally to the brain stem trigeminal nuclei. Activation of such prejunctional receptors on nerve terminals can modulate neurotransmitter release. In this context, agonists of 5-HT$_{1D}$ and 5-HT$_{1F}$ receptors are ideally placed, peripherally (see 2) to inhibit activated trigeminal nerves and promote normalization of blood vessel caliber (by preventing the release of vasoactive neuropeptides) and centrally (see 3) to intercept pain signal transmission from the meningeal blood vessels to second-order sensory neurons in the trigeminal nucleus caudalis of the brain stem (see 4). Adapted with permission from Hargreaves RJ, Shepheard SL. Pathophysiology of migraine – new insights. *Can J Neurol Sci* 1999;26(Suppl 3):S12–19

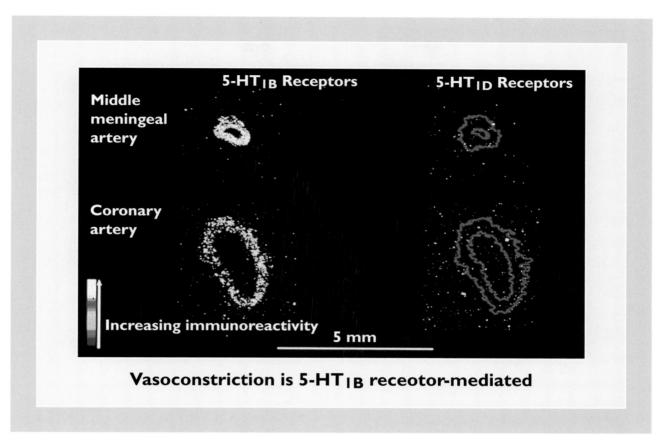

Figure 5.13 5-HT$_{1B/1D}$ receptor immunoreactivity in human cranial and coronary arteries. The left column reveals positive immunofluorescence consistent with the presence of 5-HT$_{1B}$ receptors on the blood vessels, while the right column shows negative staining for 5-HT$_{1D}$ receptors. Therefore, it is the agonist effect at 5-HT$_{1B}$ receptors that results in vasoconstriction. Reproduced with permission from Longmore J, Razzaque Z, Shaw D, *et al*. Comparison of the vasoconstrictor effects of rizatriptan and sumatriptan in human isolated cranial arteries: immunohistochemical demonstration of the involvement of 5-HT$_{1B}$ receptors. *Br J Clin Pharmacol* 1998;46:577–82

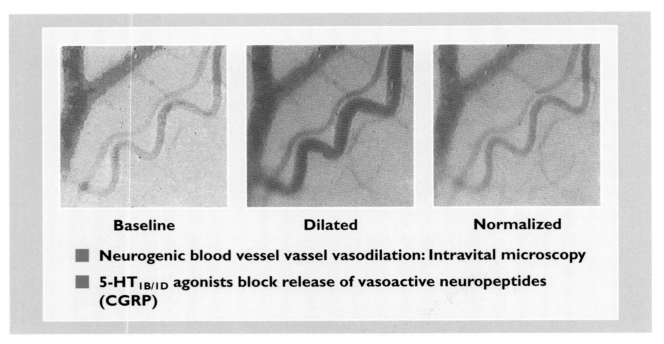

Baseline   Dilated   Normalized

■ Neurogenic blood vessel vassel vasodilation: Intravital microscopy

■ 5-HT$_{1B/1D}$ agonists block release of vasoactive neuropeptides (CGRP)

Figure 5.14 Results from a preclinical intravital microscope dural plasma protein extravasation (DPPE) assay that was used to investigate the anti-migraine action of rizatriptan. These videoframes show a branch of the middle meningeal artery embedded within the dura mater (running bottom left to top right of each section). The sequence shows the artery at baseline (left panel), in a dilated state after electrically evoked vasoactive neuropeptide release from the perivascular nerves (middle panel) and when normalized by drug treatment.

These intravital studies showed that rizatriptan blocks the electrically evoked release of peptides including CGRP from perivascular sensory nerves in the meninges but does not inhibit vessel dilation to CGRP when it is given intravenously. This suggests that rizatriptan is not a CGRP receptor antagonist but instead inhibits the release of CGRP from trigeminal sensory nerves. This blockade of neuropeptide release is thought to occur through stimulation of prejunctional 5-HT$_{1D}$ receptors. Since all of the 5-HT$_{1B/1D}$ agonists are capable of blocking the release of vasoactive neuropeptides, it suggests that one mechanism of action of these drugs is blockade of neurogenic inflammation. Reproduced with permission from Shepheard SL, Williamson DJ, Hargreaves RJ. Intravital microscope studies of dural blood vessels in rats. In: *Migraine and Headache Pathophysiology*, 1st edn. London: Martin Dunitz, 1999:103–17

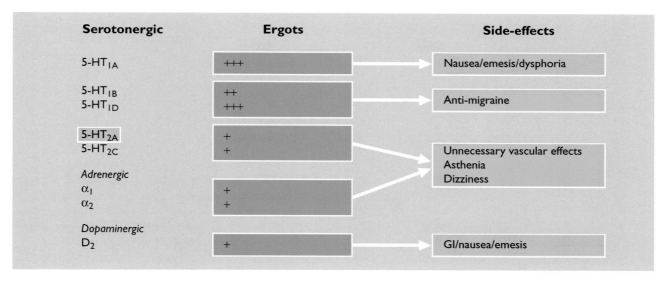

Figure 5.15 The ergots were the first 5-HT agonists used for the treatment of migraine. They are not particularly useful when given orally due to their unpredictable absorption and their low bioavailability. This is improved, however, by intranasal or rectal administration. The peripheral vascular effects of the ergots were already known during the Middle Ages, when they caused the disorder known as 'Saint Anthony's fire' due to the ingestion of bread infected by *Claviceps purpurea*, the ergot-producing fungus (see Chapter 1). This caused such a profound vasoconstriction of the extremities that patients felt as if their extremities were burning with the latter eventually turning black. The victims looked as if they had been charred by fire and the epidemic got its name from this fact. Nausea and dizziness, the common side-effects of ergots, may be explained by the actions of these compounds on multiple monoamine receptors.

Ergots are potent agonists at the 5-HT$_{1B/1D}$ receptors and this explains their anti-migraine effect. They also act on 5-HT$_{1A}$ receptors, an activation that is probably responsible for the production of nausea and dysphoria. The constriction of the peripheral vasculature is probably through activation of α-adrenoreceptors and 5-HT$_{2A}$ receptors. Agonist activity at dopamine D$_2$ receptors produces gastrointestinal disturbances, nausea and emesis. Thus, based on their pharmacologic activity at monoamine receptors, it is possible to conclude that although ergots are good anti-migraine agents, they also have many other unwanted effects. Adapted from Goadsby PJ. Serotonin 5-HT$_{1B/1D}$ receptor antagonists in migraine. *CNS Drugs* 1998;10:271–86

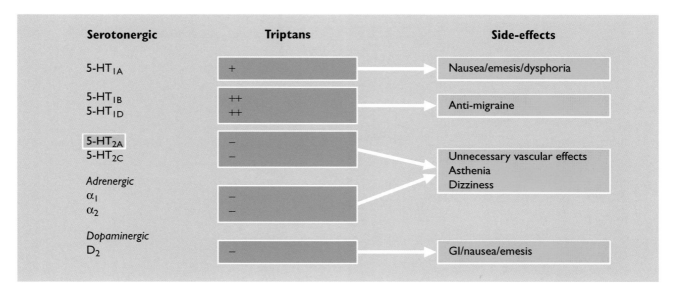

Figure 5.16 The triptans selectively target and activate 5-HT$_{1B}$ and 5-HT$_{1D}$ receptors. Like the ergots, they have potent activity at the 'anti-migraine' 5-HT$_{1B/1D}$ receptors but have much weaker action at 5-HT$_{1A}$ receptors. The triptans lack binding activity on the monoamine receptors of the ergots. Adapted from Goadsby PJ. Serotonin 5-HT$_{1B/1D}$ receptor antagonists in migraine. *CNS Drugs* 1998;10:271–86

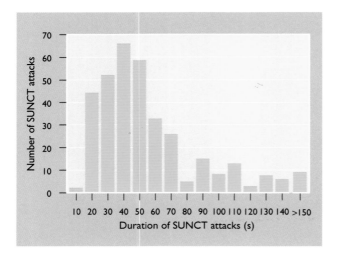

Figure 6.1 SUNCT is marked by very short lasting attacks (5 to 250 s) of headache and associated autonomic symptoms. Adapted with permission from Pareja JA, Shen JM, Kruszewski P, et al. SUNCT syndrome: duration, frequency, and temporal distribution of attacks. *Headache* 1996;36:161–5

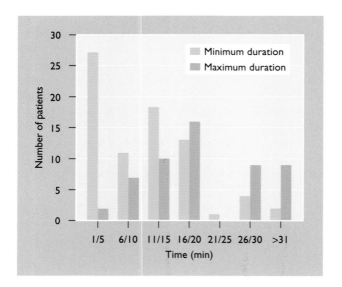

Figure 6.2 Duration of individual attacks of chronic paroxysmal hemicrania (CPH) in minutes. Most attacks will be 15 to 20 min in duration. Adapted with permission from Antonaci F, Sjaastad O. Chronic paroxysmal hemicrania (CPH): a review of the clinical manifestations. *Headache* 1989;29: 648–56

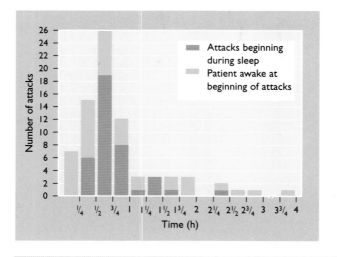

Figure 6.3 Duration of cluster attacks. Typical attack duration is 1 h or less. Adapted with permission from Russell D. Cluster headache: Severity and temporal profiles of attacks and patient activity prior to and during attacks. *Cephalalgia* 1981;1:209–16

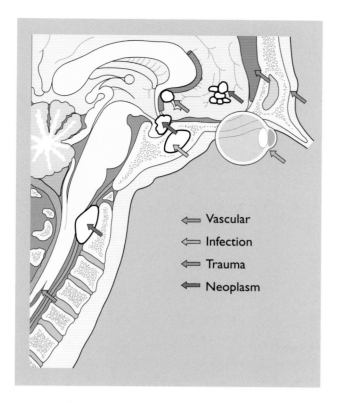

Vascular

Infection

Trauma

Neoplasm

Figure 6.4 Cluster headache is considered a primary headache disorder, so there are no underlying secondary causes. In rare instances cluster headache has been linked to various secondary causes including: aneurysms, head trauma, orbital enucleation, sphenoid sinusitis, parasellar tumors, cervical cord mengiomas or infarction, subdural hematomas and arteriovenous malformations. Adapted from the Neurology Ambassador Program with permission from the American Headache Society

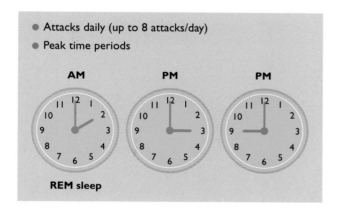

Figure 6.5 Cluster headache has a distinct circadian periodicity to its attacks. Cluster patients will get attacks at the same time each day and cluster periods at the same time each year. This suggests that the hypothalamus (suprachiasmatic nucleus) or circadian clock is playing a role in cluster genesis. A hallmark of cluster is for the patient to awaken with a cluster headache 1.5 to 2 h after falling asleep (first REM period of the night); typically these night-time attacks are the most painful. Adapted from the Neurology Ambassador Program with permission from the American Headache Society

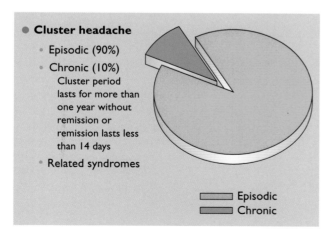

Figure 6.6 Most cluster patients have the episodic subtype so they will have periods of remission sometimes for years at a time. Adapted from the Neurology Ambassador Program with permission from the American Headache Society

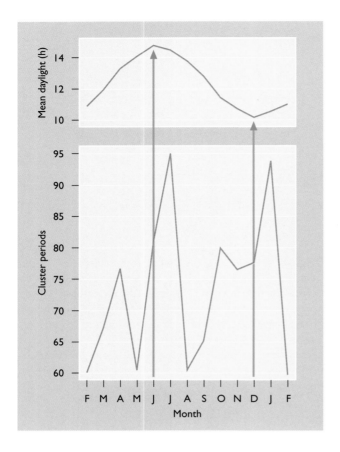

Figure 6.7 Cluster periods plotted against month of the year and mean monthly daylight duration. Cluster periods appear to occur during the longest and shortest days of the years. Adapted with permission from Kudrow L. The cyclic relationship of natural illumination to cluster period frequency. *Cephalalgia* 1987;7(Suppl 6):76–8

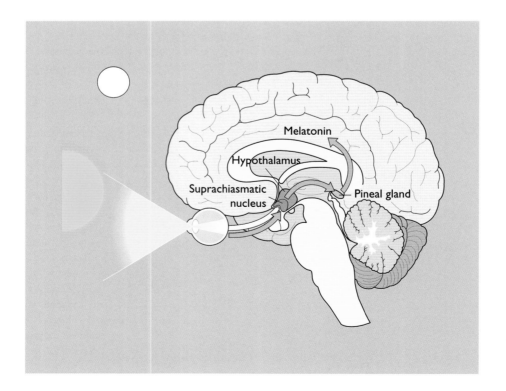

Figure 6.8 The hypothalamus or circadian clock must be involved in cluster genesis. Cluster headaches have a circannual and circadian rhythmicity, a seasonal predilection for cluster periods and there is altered secretion of hypothalamic hormones in cluster patients (testosterone, melatonin). Adapted from the Neurology Ambassador Program with permission from the American Headache Society

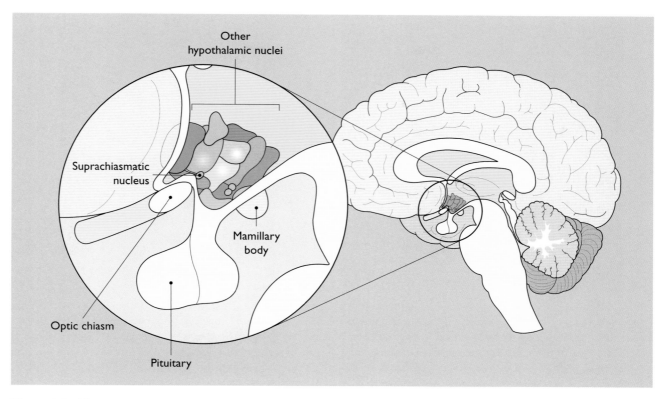

Figure 6.9   The suprachiasmatic nucleus is the human circadian clock

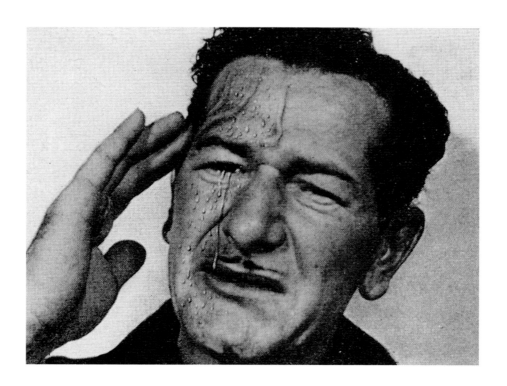

Figure 6.10   An actual cluster patient of Bayard T. Horton. Horton is considered the 'father of cluster headache'; not only did he describe the cardinal features of cluster headache but he was also the first to use oxygen in its therapy. The image shows a male undergoing a right-sided cluster headache with associated autonomic symptoms. The patient has some of the typical 'leonine facies' features recognized in cluster headache: deep nasolabial folds, peau d'orange skin and squared jaw. Reproduced with permission from Horton BT. The use of histamine in the treatment of specific types of headaches. *JAMA* 1941;116:377–83

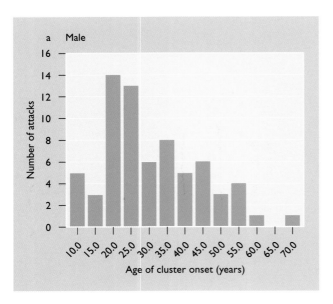
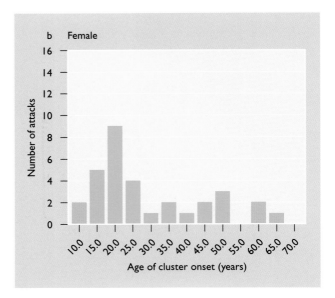

Figure 6.11 Age of cluster onset. (a) Most men develop their first ever cluster attack in their twenties or thirties (standard deviation = 13.47, mean = 31.3, n = 69); (b) women with cluster headaches have two age peaks of cluster onset (unlike men), one in their late teens or twenties and a second when they are 50 or 60 years of age (standard deviation = 15.89, mean = 29.4, n = 32). Late age of onset of female cluster headaches needs to be recognized by the treating physician. Adapted from Rozen TD, Niknam RM, Shechter AL, et al. Cluster headache in women: clinical characteristics and comparison with cluster headache in men. *J Neurol Neurosurg Psychiatr* 2001;70:613–7, with permission from the BMJ Publishing Group

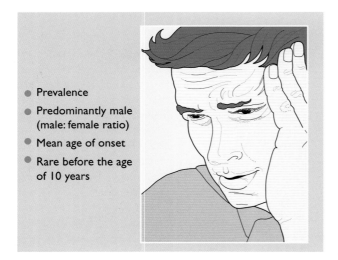

Figure 6.12 Cluster predominantly occurs in men, although more women are being diagnosed with cluster headache. The prevalence of cluster headache is 0.4% of the population. Adapted from the Neurology Ambassador Program with permission from the American Headache Society

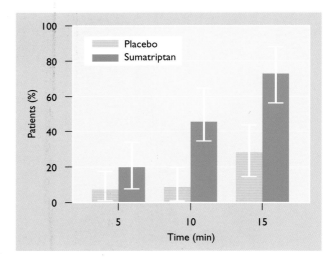

Figure 6.13 Reduction in pain severity after administration of sumatriptan injectable to patients with cluster headache. A significant response was observed by 10 and 15 min versus placebo. Adapted with permission from Olesen J, Tfelt-Hansen P, Welch KMA, eds. *The Headaches,* 2nd edn. Philadelphia, PA: Lippincott Williams & Wilkins, 2000:733

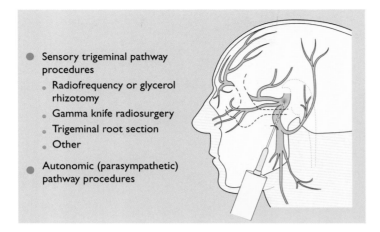

- Sensory trigeminal pathway procedures
  - Radiofrequency or glycerol rhizotomy
  - Gamma knife radiosurgery
  - Trigeminal root section
  - Other
- Autonomic (parasympathetic) pathway procedures

Figure 6.14 Presently the most effective surgical therapy for cluster is radiofrequency lesioning of the gasserian (trigeminal) ganglion. Under radiographic control a device is inserted into the cheek and directed through the foramen ovale into the area of the gasserian ganglion where a specific denervating agent (radiofrequency, glycerol) is then used. Adapted from the Neurology Ambassador Program with permission from the American Headache Society

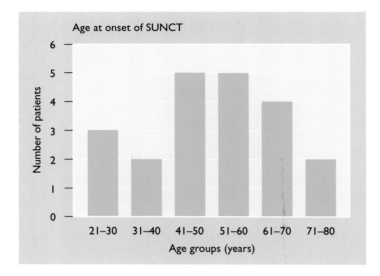

Figure 6.15 SUNCT is considered a disorder of the elderly, although there are some reported cases younger than age 40. Adapted with permission from Pareja JA, Sjaastad O. SUNCT syndrome. A clinical review. *Headache* 1997;37:195–202

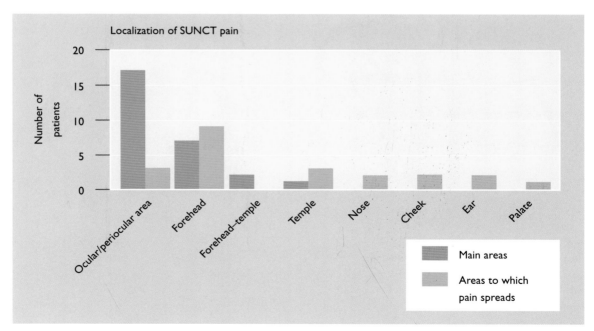

Figure 6.16 SUNCT pain is located in or around the eye and/or the forehead region. It can spread to extra-trigeminal innervated areas. Adapted with permission from Pareja JA, Sjaastad O. SUNCT syndrome. A clinical review. *Headache* 1997;37:195–202

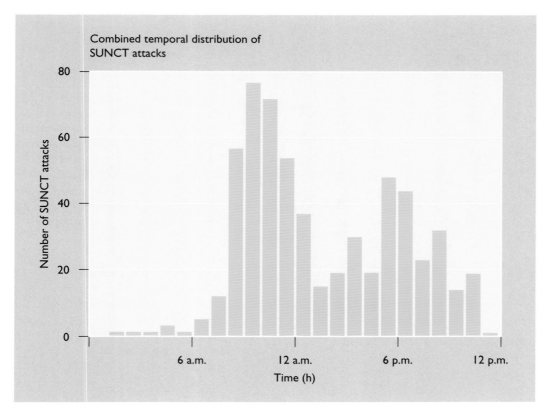

Figure 6.17 SUNCT attacks tend to cluster around morning and afternoon/evening times, although attacks can occur at any time during the day. Adapted with permission from Pareja JA, Shen JM, Kruszewski P, *et al*. SUNCT syndrome: duration, frequency, and temporal distribution of attacks. *Headache* 1996;36:161–5

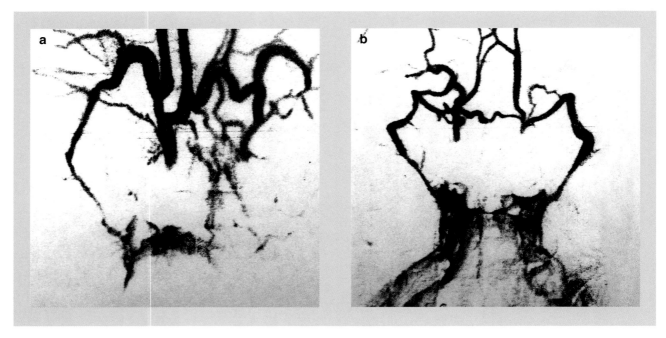

Figure 6.18 (a) Orbital phlebogram showing narrowing of the superior ophthalmic vein and partial occlusion of the cavernous sinus in an episodic cluster patient; (b) normal phlebogram for comparison. Reproduced with permission from Hannerz J, Ericson K, Bergstrand G. Orbital phlebography in patients with cluster headache. *Cephalalgia* 1987;7:207–11

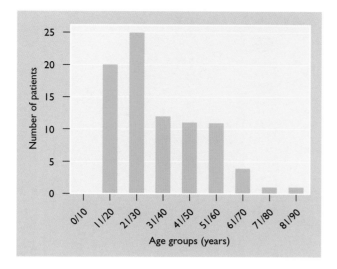

Figure 6.19 Chronic paroxysmal hemicrania (CPH) typically starts to occur in the teens or twenties, very similar to the age of onset of cluster. Adapted with permission from Antonaci F, Sjaastad O. Chronic paroxysmal hemicrania (CPH): a review of the clinical manifestations. *Headache* 1989;29: 648–56

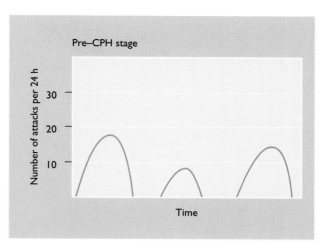

Figure 6.21 The natural history of chronic paroxysmal hemicrania (CPH) is unknown. When Sjaastad first identified CPH he noticed that some patients went through a pre-CPH stage of CPH attacks with remission periods. In some patients these patients never went on to have CPH. Most likely this pre-CPH stage is episodic paroxysmal hemicrania (EPH). Adapted with permission from Russell D, Sjaastad O. Chronic paroxysmal hemicrania. In: Pfaffenrath V, Sjaastad O, Lundberg PO, eds. *Updating in Headache*. Berlin: Springer-Verlag, 1984:1–6, copyright © Springer-Verlag

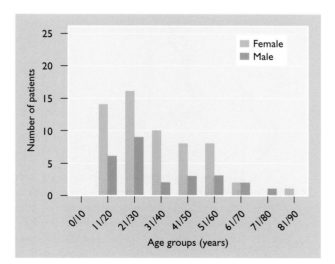

Figure 6.20 Both females and males who develop chronic paroxysmal hemicrania (CPH) typically have their first attacks in their teens or twenties. Adapted with permission from Antonaci F, Sjaastad O. Chronic paroxysmal hemicrania (CPH): a review of the clinical manifestations. *Headache* 1989;29: 648–56

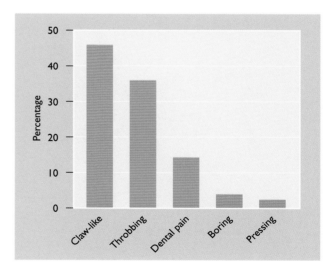

Figure 6.22 Quality of chronic paroxysmal hemicrania (CPH) pain. Adapted with permission from Antonaci F, Sjaastad O. Chronic paroxysmal hemicrania (CPH): a review of the clinical manifestations. *Headache* 1989;29:648–56

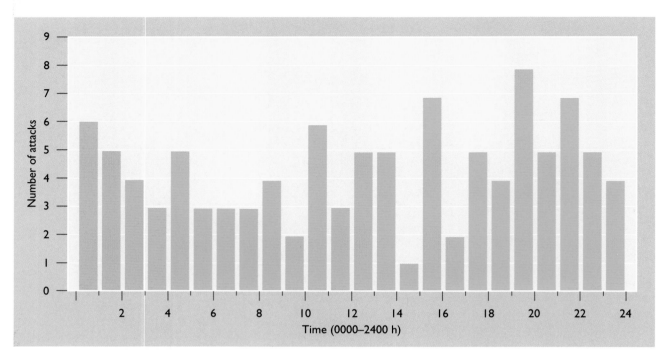

Figure 6.23 Chronic paroxysmal hemicrania attacks, unlike cluster attacks, occur anytime during the day and night and do not have a predeliction for nocturnal attacks. Adapted with permission from Russell D. Chronic paroxysmal hemicrania: severity, duration and time of occurrence of attacks. *Cephalalgia* 1984;4:53–6

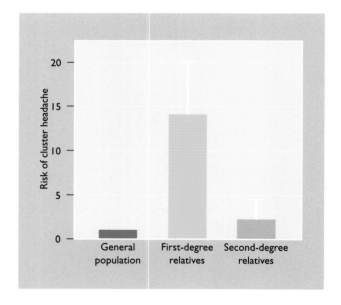

Figure 6.24 Cluster is not considered to have a genetic predisposition as is seen in migraine, but first-degree relatives have a 14-fold increased risk of developing cluster headaches in their lifetime. Adapted with permission from Olesen J, Tfelt-Hansen P, Welch KMA, eds. *The Headaches*, 2nd edn. Philadelphia, PA: Lippincott Williams & Wilkins, 2000:680

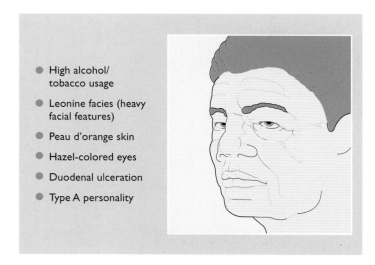

- High alcohol/ tobacco usage
- Leonine facies (heavy facial features)
- Peau d'orange skin
- Hazel-colored eyes
- Duodenal ulceration
- Type A personality

Figure 6.25 Cluster headache has been linked to a typical facies, eye color and certain medical conditions. Adapted from the Neurology Ambassador Program with permission from the American Headache Society

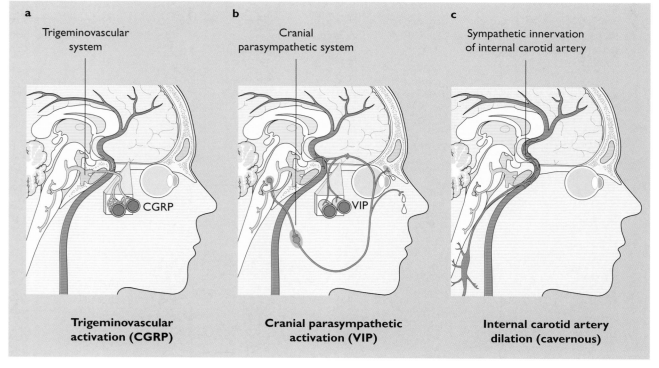

a
Trigeminovascular system

b
Cranial parasympathetic system

c
Sympathetic innervation of internal carotid artery

Trigeminovascular activation (CGRP)

Cranial parasympathetic activation (VIP)

Internal carotid artery dilation (cavernous)

Figure 6.26 The true pathogenesis of cluster headache is still unknown. What must be accounted for when determining a unified theory of cluster pathogenesis are: (a) The pain is orbital in location. This means the ipsilateral sensory trigeminal nerve system is involved. Trigeminal afferents transmit cephalic pain via the ophthalmic division of the trigeminal nerve synapse in the trigeminal ganglion which then relays this sensory input to the trigeminal nucleus caudalis in the brainstem. Calcitonin gene-related peptide (CGRP) is the neurotransmitter released in this system; (b) Ipsilateral symptoms of parasympathetic activation (lacrimation, nasal congestion). Cranial parasympathetic innervation of the intracranial vessels arise in primary order neurons in the superior salivatory nucleus in the pons. Efferents from this system (via the seventh cranial nerve) act to stimulate the nasal and lacrimal glands. Vasoactive intestinal peptide (VIP) is a marker of activation of the cranial parasympathetic system; (c) Ipsilateral symptoms of sympathetic dysfunction (miosis, ptosis, partial Horner's syndrome). As a result of activation of sensory trigeminal and cranial parasympathetic systems there is blood vessel dilation in the internal carotid artery. If the cavernous carotid artery (level at which the parasympathetic, sympathetic and trigeminal fibers converge) dilates, it can cause compression of the sympathetic system with the production of a postganglionic Horner's syndrome. Adapted from the Neurology Ambassador Program with permission from the American Headache Society

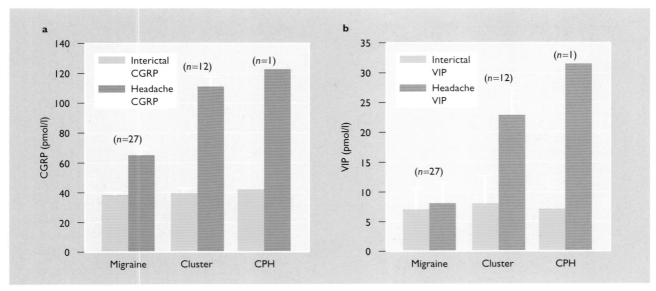

Figure 6.27 Changes in calcitonin gene-related peptide (CGRP; a) and vasoactive intestinal polypeptide (VIP; b) levels during migraine, cluster and chronic paroxysmal hemicrania (CPH) attacks. Note elevation of both CGRP and VIP levels in the trigeminal-autonomic cephalgia (TAC) headaches but not in migraine. Adapted from Goadsby PJ, Lipton RB. A review of paroxysmal hemicranias, SUNCT syndrome and other short-lasting headaches with autonomic feature, including new cases. *Brain* 1997;120:193–209, with permission by Oxford University Press

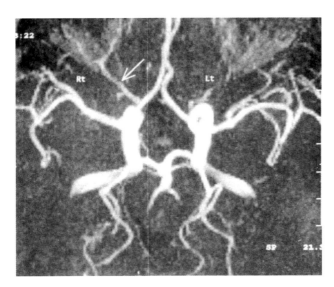

Figure 6.28 Dilation of the ophthalmic artery during a spontaneous cluster attack. The artery normalized after cluster remission. Artery dilation in cluster headache may result from trigeminal nerve activation with release of calcitonin gene-related peptide (CGRP) or from an inflammatory process in the cavernous sinus and tributary veins leading to venous stasis and resultant artery dilation. Vascular congestion within the cavernous sinus region can explain the pain of cluster and the sympathetic damage seen during attacks. A venous vasculitis theory for cluster is another possible etiology for cluster pathogenesis. Reproduced with permission from Waldenlind E, Ekbom K, Torhall J. MR-angiography during spontaneous attacks of cluster headache: a case report. *Headache* 1993;33:291–5

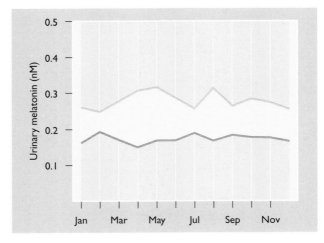

Figure 6.29 Urine melatonin levels were examined for up to 14 months in episodic cluster headache patients (red line) and healthy controls (yellow line). The mean levels of urinary melatonin were significantly lower in patients than controls in both cluster periods and during remissions. Adapted from Waldenlind E, Gustafsson SA, Ekbom K, Wetterberg L. Circadian secretion of cortisol and melatonin in cluster headache during active cluster periods and remission. *J Neurol Neurosurg Psychiatr* 1987;50:207–13, with permission by the BMJ Publishing Group

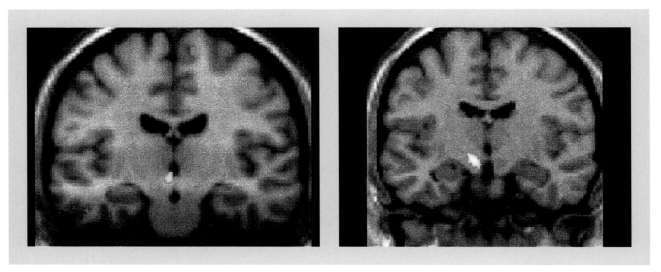

Figure 6.30 Image on the left demonstrates hypothalamic activation during a cluster attack on PET. The image on the right is a voxel-based morphometric analysis of the structural T1-weighted MRI scans from 25 right-handed cluster patients revealing a significant difference in hypothalamic gray matter density (yellow) compared with non-cluster patients. The hypothalamus of cluster patients appears to have an increased volume compared with controls. Adapted from the Neurology Ambassador Program with permission from the American Headache Society

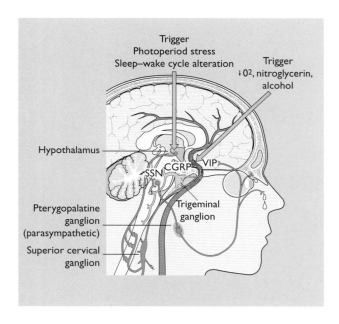

Figure 6.31 Image showing how the hypothalamus, trigeminal sensory, cranial parasympathetic and carotid sympathetic systems interact to produce a cluster headache. The brainstem connection between the trigeminal and cranial sympathetic systems (trigeminal-autonomic reflex pathway) helps to explain the clinical phenotype of the trigeminal-autonomic cephalgias (TACs). CGRP, calcitonin gene-related peptide; SSN, superior salivatory nucleus; VIP, vasoactive intestinal polypeptide. Adapted from the Neurology Ambassador Program with permission from the American Headache Society

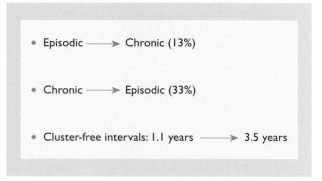

Figure 6.32 The natural history of cluster headaches is not well documented in the literature. About 13% of episodic cluster patients will develop into chronic cluster, whereas one-third of chronic patients will change to episodic cluster. Being on a preventive appears to help with the latter transition. Most cluster patients will continue over their lifetime to have the same number of attacks per day and the same duration for each attack. Adapted from the Neurology Ambassador Program with permission from the American Headache Society

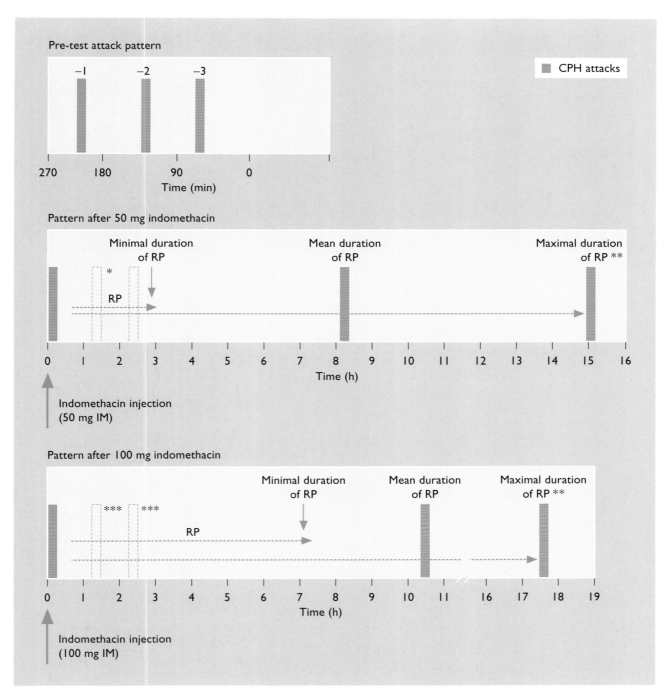

Figure 6.33 Indomethacin is the sole treatment of choice in chronic paroxysmal hemicrania (CPH). Antonaci *et al.* have described the 'indotest' in which a 50 mg indomethacin IM test dosage can be given to patients in the office with possible CPH. When looking at the mean interval of attack frequency pre-indomethacin and post-indomethacin, after indomethacin the attack frequency is reduced (refractory period (RP) was initiated post-indomethacin). If a patient after indomethacin does not get their typical next attack, then indomethacin should be effective in that patient for their headaches. *Hatched lines indicate putative attacks that have not materialized; **pre-attack pattern re-established in all patients; ***the timing of the anticipated attacks is not based on exact recording of the attack pattern prior to the 100 mg test. Adapted with permission from Antonaci F, Pareja JA, Caminero AB, Sjaastad O. Chronic paroxysmal hemicrania and hemicrania continua. Parenteral indomethacin: the 'indotest'. *Headache* 1998;38:122–8

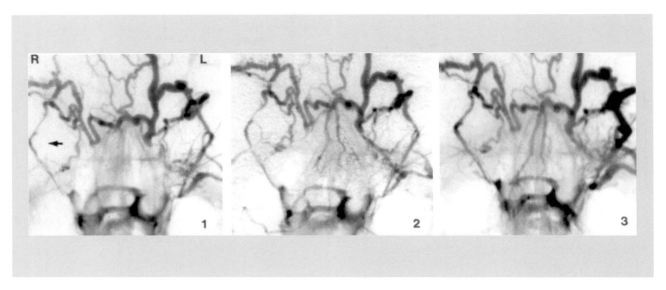

Figure 6.34 Orbital phlebography in a 49-year-old man with SUNCT. On the side of the pain on the right (see arrow), there was narrowing of the whole superior ophthalmic vein (1 and 2). Orbital phlebography completed when the patient was in a remission state was normal (3). The findings suggest that SUNCT, at least in a subset of patients, may be caused by a venous vasculitis. Reproduced with permission from Hannerz J, Greitz D, Hansson P, Ericson K. SUNCT may be another manifestation of orbital venous vasculitis. *Headache* 1992;32:384–9

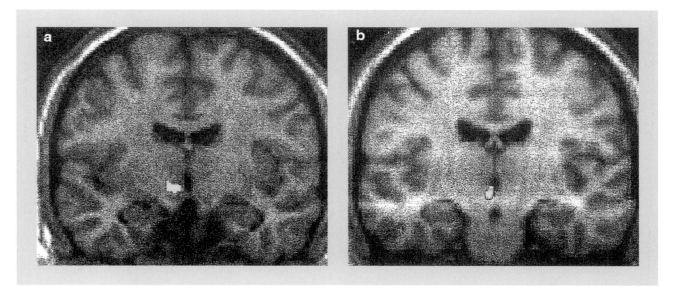

Figure 6.35 BOLD contrast-MRI of the brain of a 71-year-old woman with SUNCT syndrome. (a) Activation is noted in the ipsilateral posterior hypothalamic gray region (yellow). Almost the same exact area of activation is noted during a cluster attack (b) suggesting a similar underlying cause of these clinically disparate TACs. Adapted with permission from May A, Bahra A, Buchel C, et al. Functional magnetic resonance imaging in spontaneous attacks of SUNCT: Short-lasting neuralgiform headache with conjunctival injection and tearing. *Ann Neurol* 1999;46:791–4, copyright © John Wiley & Sons, Inc

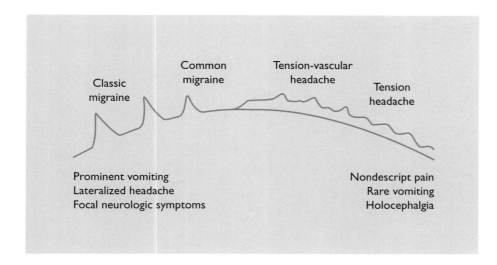

Figure 7.1 'The continuum of benign recurring headache' was introduced by Raskin. Adapted with permission from Raskin NH. *Headache*, 2nd edn. New York: Churchill Livingstone, 1988:215–24

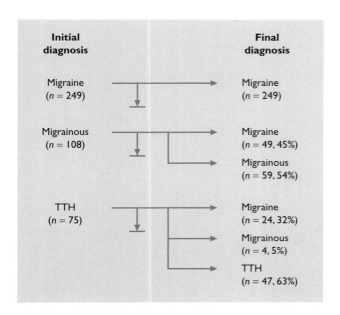

Figure 7.2 Reclassification of headache diagnosis based on diary review. TTH, tension-type headache. Adapted from Lipton RB, Stewart WF, Hall C, *et al.* The misdiagnosis of disabling episodic headache: Results from the Spectrum Study. Presented at the International Headache Congress, June 2001

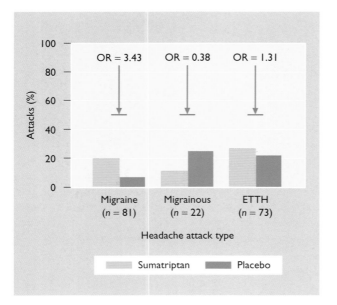

Figure 7.3 Pain-free response at 2 h by headache attack type in individuals with an initial diagnosis of tension-type headache and a final diagnosis of migraine. ETTH, episodic tension-type headache; OR, odds ratio. Adapted with kind permission of Richard B. Lipton

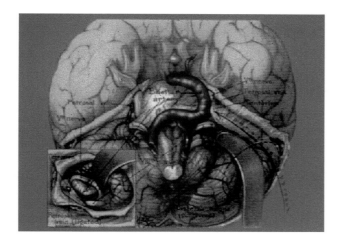

Figure 8.1 Vascular compression theory for trigeminal neuralgia. One of the first surgical proponents of the vascular theory was Walter Dandy. In 1934, Dandy wrote, 'I believe no less responsible for the production of trigeminal neuralgia; these are the arteries and veins which impinge upon and frequently distort the sensory root. In the region of the sensory root the superior arterial branch forms a loop…as the artery hardens from advancing age, the nerve becomes indented by the arterial branch'. Reproduced from Dandy WE. Concerning the cause of trigeminal neuralgia. *Am J Surg* 1934;24:447–55, with permission from Excerpta Medica Inc

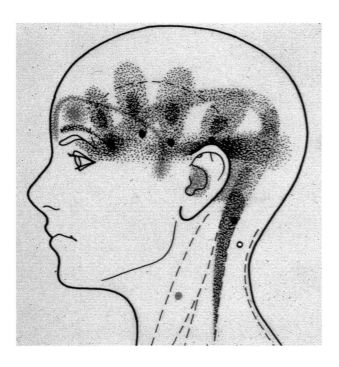

Figure 8.2 Overlapping pain referral patterns from myofascial trigger points in various masticatory and cervical muscles produce typical unilateral or bilateral migraine or tension-type headache. Reproduced with kind permission of Bernadette Jaeger

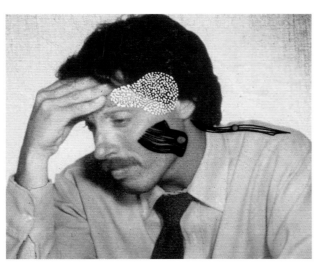

Figure 8.3 Referred pain from superficial masseter and upper trapezius myofascial trigger points may produce unilateral or bilateral tension-type and migraine headache symptoms. Reproduced with kind permission of Bernadette Jaeger

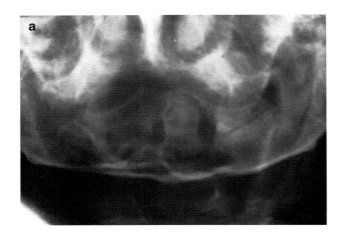

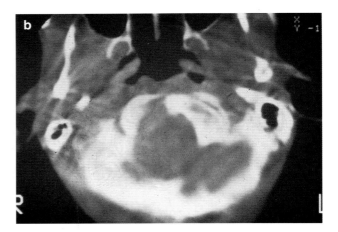

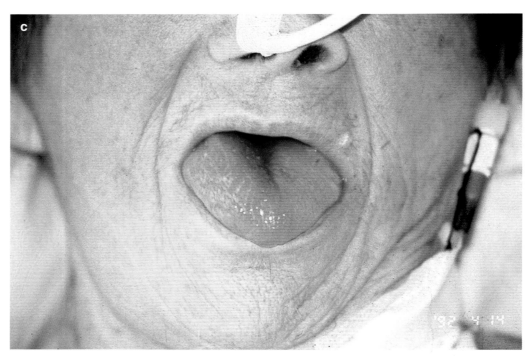

Figure 8.4 (a), (b) and (c) belong to the same patient, a 67-year-old woman with severe, continuous left occipital pain and swallowing difficulties during the previous two weeks. The pain became unbearable with right suboccipital palpation or on neck rotation to the left. Neurologic examination showed a right twelfth nerve paralysis. She died suddenly several days after admission. Clinical diagnosis was 'right occipital condyle syndrome' secondary to a metastasis of unknown origin. (a) Posteroanterior skull radiograph with an inclination of 30° showing an osteolytic lesion of the right occipital condyle; (b) axial skull base. CT scan with bone window setting showing erosion of the right occipital condyle; (c) right hypoglossal paralysis. Reproduced with permission from Moris G, Roig C, Misiego M, *et al.* The distinctive headache of the occipital condyle syndrome: A report of four cases. *Headache* 1998;38:308–11

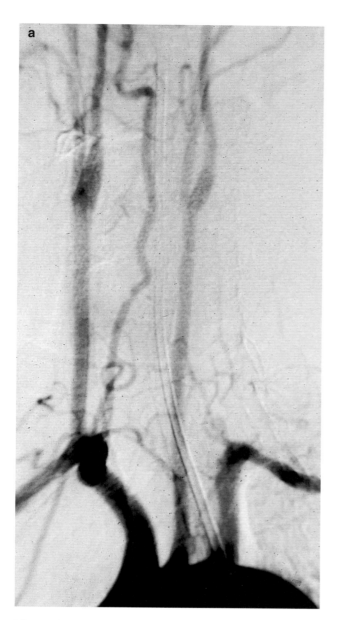

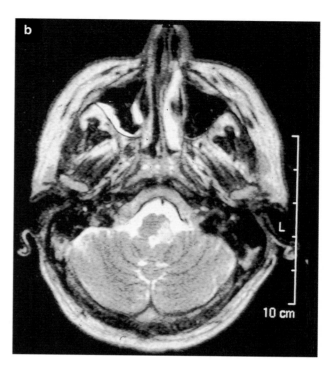

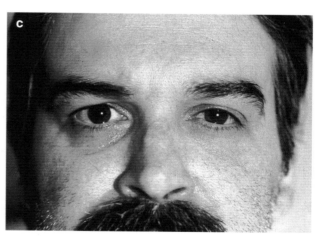

Figure 8.5 (a), (b) and (c) are from the same patient, a 37-year-old with a Wallenberg's syndrome accompanied by retro-ocular headache with autonomic features resembling 'continuous' cluster headache. This case suggests that all the symptomatology typical of cluster headache can be secondary to a pure central lesion. (a) Angiography showing an occlusion of the left vertebral artery, with no sign of dissection; (b) T2-weighted MRI showing an infarct of the left posterior inferior cerebellar artery (PICA) territory; (c) close-up picture of the patient's face showing left palpebral ptosis and conjunctival injection. Reproduced from Cid C, Berciano J, Pascual J. Retro-ocular headache with autonomic features resembling 'continuous' cluster headache in lateral medullary infarction. *J Neurol Neurosurg Psychiatr* 2000;69:134–41, with permission by the BMJ Publishing Group

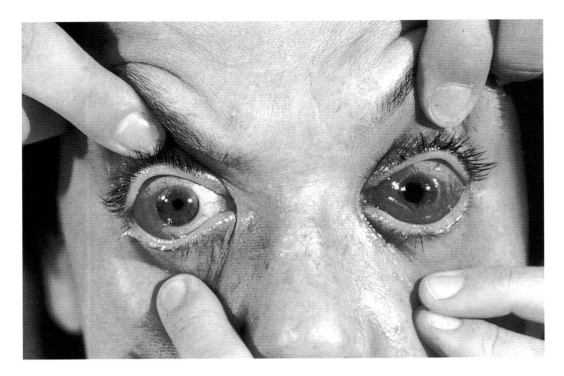

Figure 8.6 Very severe conjunctival injection (more pronounced in the patient's left side) and uveitis in a 63-year-old woman presenting as bilateral periocular headache as the first sign of a confirmed Wegener's syndrome. Headache and ocular manifestations resolved after aggressive treatment with steroids and cyclophosphamide. Reproduced with kind permission of Julio Pascual

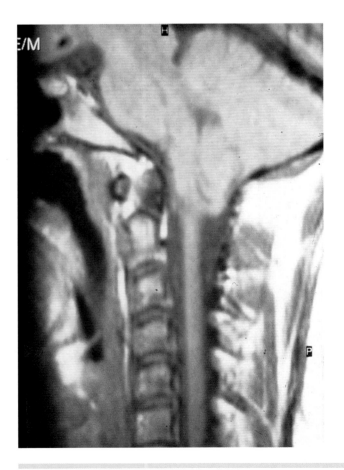

Figure 8.7 Cranio-cervical MRI study of a 39-year-old-woman complaining of brief (second–1 minute) occipital headache when coughing and other Valsalva maneuvers showing tonsillar descent. Sagittal MRI T1 W1 pulse sequence demonstrates low lying tonsils, normal fourth ventricle and normal posterior fossae anatomy indicative of Chiari 1. Headache has disappeared after suboccipital craniectomy. Reproduced with permission from Pascual J, Iglesias F, Oterino A, et al. Cough, exertional and sexual headache. *Neurology* 1996;46:1520–4

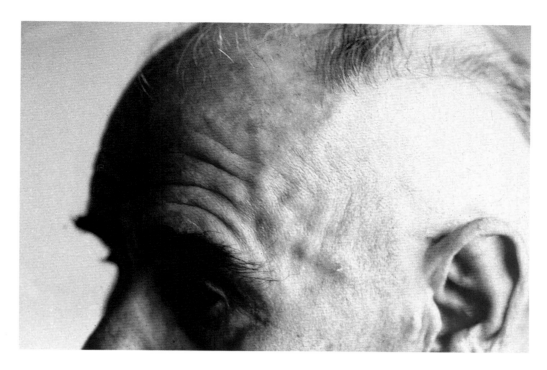

Figure 8.8 This 78-year-old man went to hospital due to constant temporal headache during the previous two months. On exami-nation there was no pulsation in the left temporal artery, which appeared thickened and painful on palpation. The erythrocyte sedi-mentation rate was 96 mm in the first hour, while a temporal artery biopsy showed changes diagnostic of giant-cell arteritis. Courtesy of José Berciano, University Hospital Marques de Valdecilla, Santander, Spain

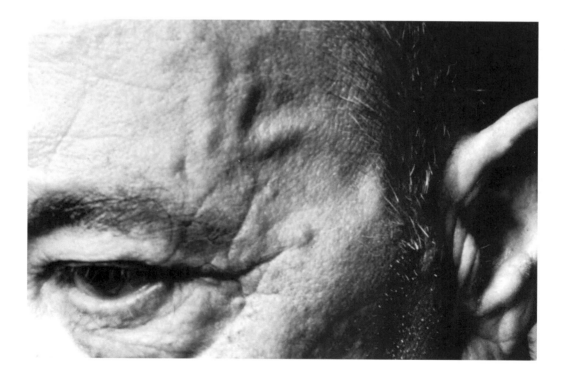

Figure 8.9 Seventy-year-old man with giant-cell arteritis. A portion of the anterior branch of the left temporal artery is visibly swollen. It was tender and thickened on palpation. Reproduced with permission from Caselli RJ, Hunder GG. Giant cell arteritis and polymyalgia rheumatica. In: Silberstein SD, Lipton RB, Dalessio DJ, eds. *Wolff's Headache and other Head Pain*, 7th edn. New York: Oxford University Press, 2001:525–35

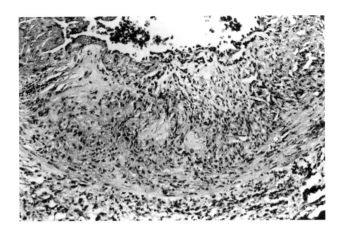

Figure 8.10 Temporal artery biopsy specimen showing active inflammation in all three vascular layers (intima, media, adventitia). The lumen is partially shown, at the top of the figure, and is narrowed. In most temporal artery biopsy specimens with giant-cell arteritis, the media, especially the inner media in the region of the internal elastic lamina, is involved to the greatest extent and the intimal and adventitial layers are involved to a lesser degree than in this patient (hematoxylin and eosin stain, 200x). Reproduced with permission from Casselli RJ, Hunder GG. Giant cell arteritis and polymyalgia rheumatica. In: Silberstein SD. Lipton RB, Dalessio DJ, eds. *Wolff's Headache and Other Head Pain*, 7th edn. New York: Oxford University Press, 2001:525–35

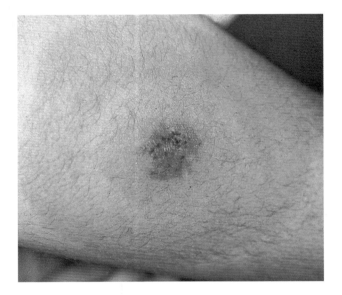

Figure 8.11 Lyme disease most often presents with a characteristic 'bull's eye' rash, erythema migrans, accompanied by non-specific symptoms such as fever, malaise, fatigue, myalgia and joint aches (arthralgia). Many patients complain of persistent daily headaches

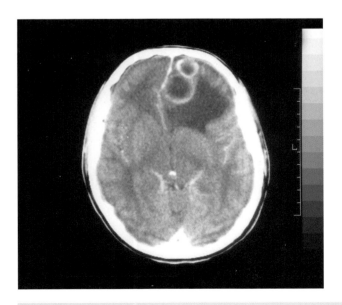

Figure 8.12 A 22-year-old man with a one-month history of a left hemicranial pain and cluster-like features. An axial CT scan post-enhancement demonstrated a multilocular lesion in the left frontal lobe with white matter edema, displacement of the falx to the right and enhancement of the rings measuring 3.5 cm at the widest. This is a pyogenic brain abscess approximately 14 days old. Reproduced with kind permission of Germany Goncalves Veloso

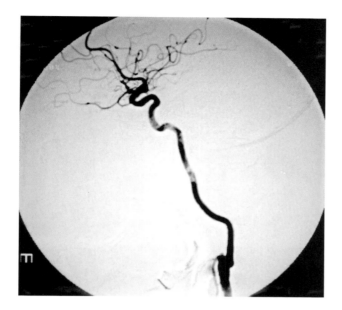

Figure 8.13 A 53-year-old female patient with a strong pain in the left periocular and temporal region. She presented with autonomic signs, eyelid ptosis and conjunctival injection, ipsilateral to and concurrent with the pain. The duration of the pain was 40 min. It occurred three times per day and was worse at night. As a result of the painful episodes she had decreased sensitivity in the left facial region. The angiogram disclosed an occlusion at the proximal region of the external carotid artery on the left. Patient experienced total relief using verapamil. Reproduced with kind permission of Vera Lucia Faria Xavier

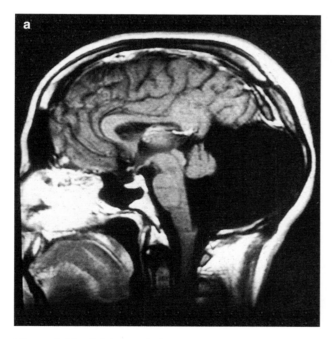

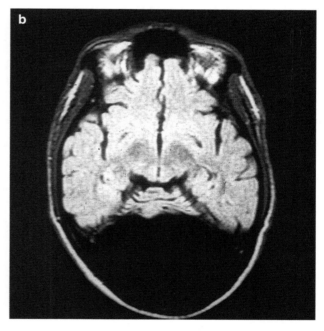

Figure 8.14 A 34-year-old healthy farmer reported a mild occipital headache for 4 weeks. The general and neurologic examinations were normal. (a) Sagittal T1 W1 MRI and (b) axial T1 W1 MRI showed a large cyst in the posterior fossa displacing the cerebellar hemispheres upwards; this is likely to be a congenital Dandy–Walker abnormality. Surgical approaches were contraindicated by the neurosurgical staff. After 3 years the patient remains asymptomatic, except for transient, mild headaches associated with emotional stress. Reproduced with kind permission of Pericles de Andrade Maranhão-Filho

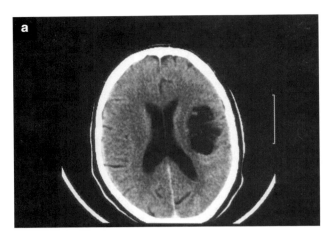
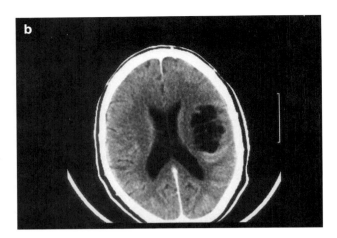

Figure 8.15 A 35-year-old man with a history of chronic daily headache and recent-onset partial motor seizures. (a) Axial CT scan shows multiloculated cysts in the left sylvian fissure; (b) axial CT scan at the same level. The subarachnoid lesion is not enhanced. The diagnosis is cysticercosis. Reproduced with kind permission of Suzana M.F. Malheiros

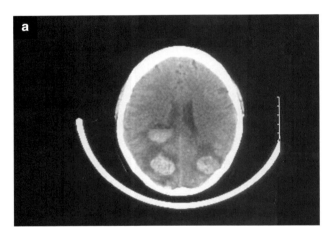
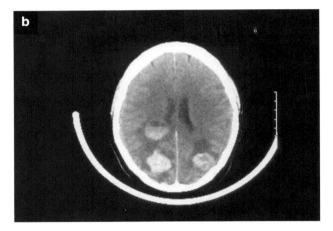

Figure 8.16 A 34-year-old woman with a history of thunderclap headache during sport activity associated with blurred vision. (a) Axial CT scan shows multifocal high-density intraparenchymal lesions; (b) CT scan shows an irregularly enhancing rim of the three lesions each located bilaterally in the parietal lobes with surrounding edema. Note a fluid–fluid level within the right periventricular lesion. The lesions were confirmed as metastatic melanoma. Reproduced with kind permission of Suzana M.F. Malheiros

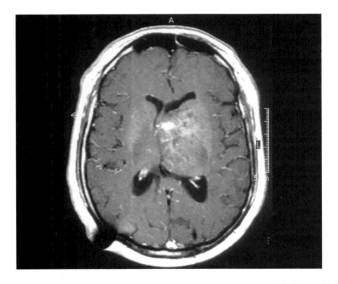

Figure 8.17 A 60-year-old man with a six-month history of pressing/tightening headache that antedated the development of mild right hemiparesis. Axial post-contrast T1-weighted MR scan shows a large, enhancing, ill-delineated left basal ganglia mass. The diagnosis is anaplastic astrocytoma. Reproduced with kind permission of Suzana M.F. Malheiros

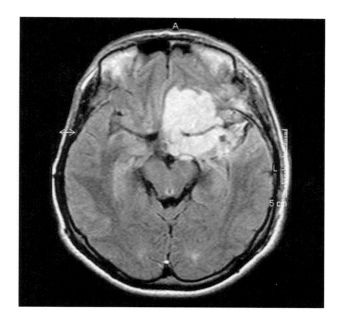

Figure 8.18 A 29-year-old man with a history of sudden-onset headache associated with exertional worsening. Axial FLAIR image demonstrates a hyperintense left fronto-temporal scallop-bordered mass (approximately 5 × 3.7 cm) well circumscribed with no edema. The diagnosis is primitive neuroendodermal tumor (PNET). Reproduced with kind permission of Suzana M.F. Malheiros

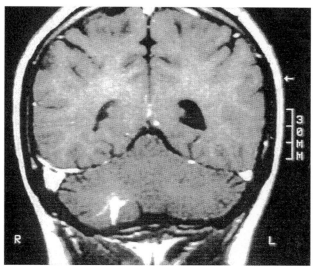

Figure 8.19 Sagittal T1 W1 MRI post-enhancement venous angioma. A right cerebellar linear enhancing structure with a trans-cerebellar course demonstrating uniform enhancement and classic umbrella shape

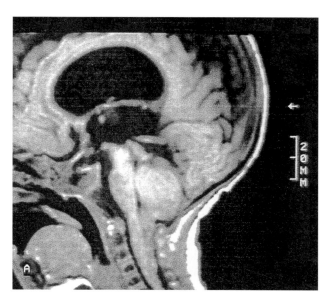

Figure 8.20 Sagittal T1 W1 non-enhanced MRI demonstrating a Chiari II malformation. Note the low-lying tonsils, flattening of the aqueduct, compression of the fourth ventricle and a widened cervical cord

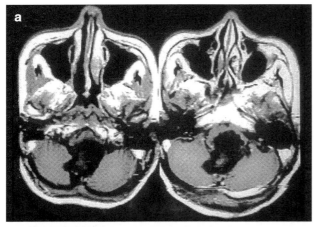

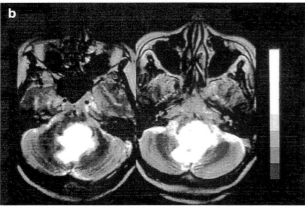

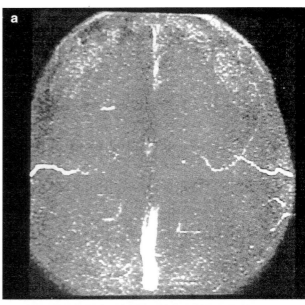

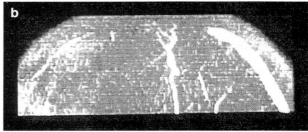

Figure 8.21 Two axial T1 WI MRI non-enhancing images reveal a large hypointense, scallop-bordered mass with extension to the foramen of Luschka, compressing the brainstem and fourth ventricle which demonstrates hyperintensity on the T2-weighted image (b) so that it becomes iso-intense with the cerebral spinal fluid (CSF)

Figure 8.23 A patient who presented with headache with papilledema. These are images demonstrating a filling defect or lack of filling of the superior sagittal sinus consistent with thrombosis

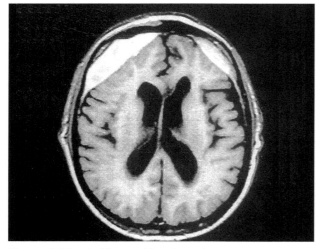

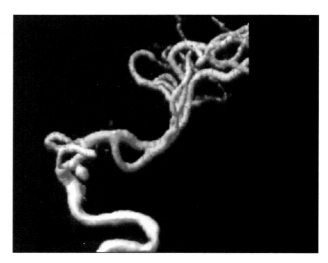

Figure 8.22 A 40-year-old male with continued headache following head trauma from a motorcycle accident. An axial T1 non-enhanced image shows bilateral, concave, hyperintense collections that are 3 days to 3 weeks old. The diagnosis is subacute subdural hematoma

Figure 8.24 Carotid arteriogram showing an aneurysm which comes to a point consistent with this being the area of pathology. No areas of spasm are noted. Reproduced with kind permission of Nitamar Abdala

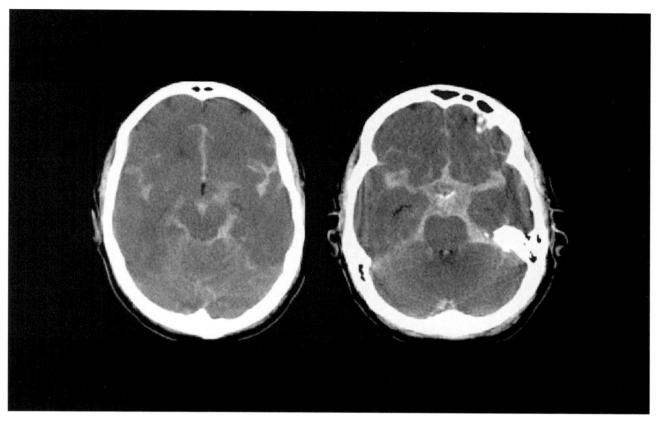

Figure 8.25 Two axial CT scans showing diffuse blood-filled CSF and cisternal spaces. There is increased density consistent with a diffuse subarachnoid hemorrhage. Reproduced with kind permission of Nitamar Abdala

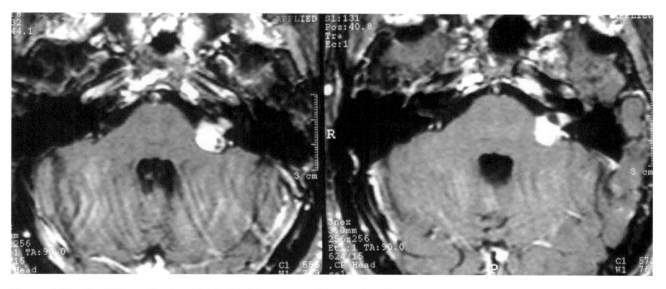

Figure 8.26 A middle-aged male with left-sided head pain and hearing loss. Two posterior fossae T1 MRI post-enhancement images show a cerebellopontine angle component of 1 cm with an intracanalicular extension. Uniformly enhancing mass with a cisternal and intracanalicular component; widening of the internal auditory canal is consistent with a vestibular schwannoma. Reproduced with kind permission of Nitamar Abdala

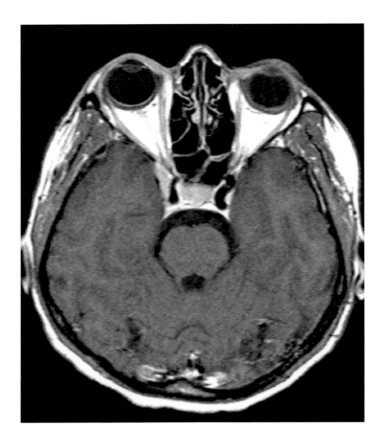

Figure 8.27 Tolosa-Hunt syndrome is an idiopathic inflammatory condition that usually presents with painful ophthalmoplegia. An axial T1 MRI shows a soft tissue mass filling the lateral aspect of the right cavernous sinus compressing and medially displacing the carotid artery and extruding to the apex of the right orbit. Reproduced with kind permission of Nitamar Abdala

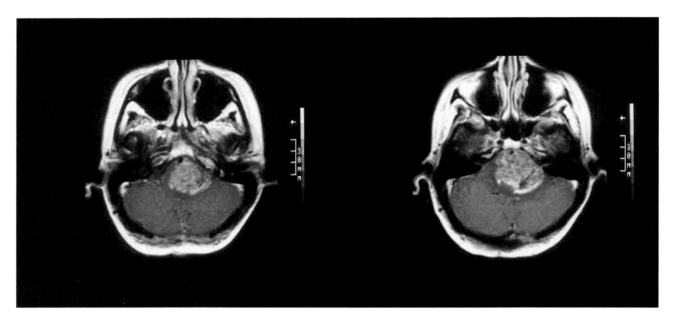

Figure 8.28 A 32-year-old woman with a four-month history of a new-onset throbbing headache followed by sixth nerve palsy and ataxia. Axial post-contrast T1-weighted MR scans show a large, enhancing, well-delineated mass that expands and distorts the pons. The diagnosis is anaplastic astrocytoma. Reproduced with kind permission of Suzana M.F. Malheiros

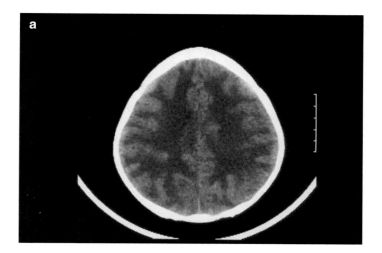

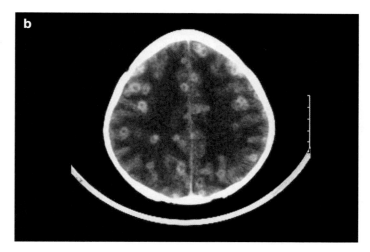

Figure 8.29 A 15-year-old girl with a history of progressive severe headache initiating 2 weeks before, associated with nausea, vomiting and decreased consciousness. (a) Axial CT scan shows ill-defined low-density changes in the white matter of both hemispheres; (b) axial CT scan at the same level shows multifocal subcortical white matter ring-enhancing lesions. The diagnosis is cysticercosis. Reproduced with kind permission of Suzana M.F. Malheiros

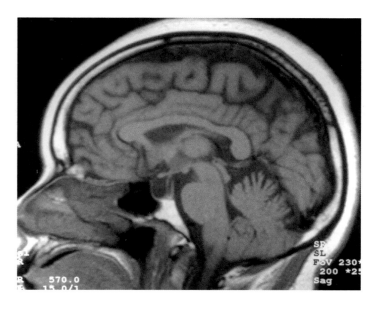

Figure 8.30 A middle-aged woman presenting with headaches is found to have an empty sella. A sagittal T1 MRI demonstrating a stretched pituitary infundibulum with no significant visible pituitary tissue

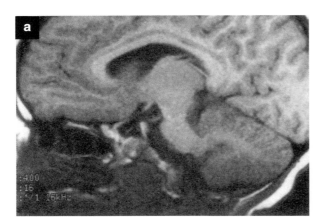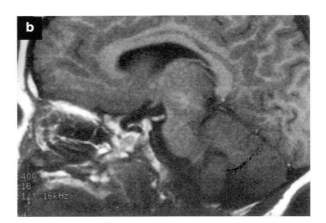

Figure 8.31 Three-year-old boy with two prior episodes of spontaneously resolving oculomotor nerve palsy. (a) and (b), sagittal T1-weighted MR images before (a) and after (b) contrast administration show diffuse thickening and enhancement of the oculomotor nerve. The symptoms resolved spontaneously in 6 weeks. Reproduced with permission from Mark AS, Casselman J, Brown D, *et al.* Ophthalmoplegic migraine: Reversible enhancement and thickening of the cisternal segment of the oculomotor nerve on contrast-enhanced MR images. *AJNR Am J Neuroradiol* 1998;19:1887–91, copyright © American Society of Neuroradiology (www.ajnr.org)

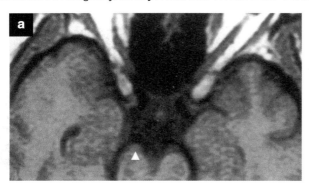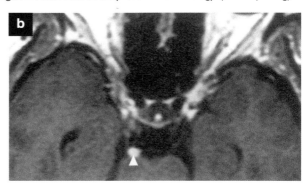

Figure 8.32 Twenty-seven-year old woman with two prior episodes of headache and oculomotor nerve palsy. (a) and (b), axial non-contrast (a) and contrast-enhanced (b) T1-weighted images show focal nodular enhancement of the exit zone of the oculomotor nerve (see arrows). Follow-up study showed virtually complete resolution of the enhancement. Reproduced with permission from Mark AS, Casselman J, Brown D, *et al.* Ophthalmoplegic migraine: Reversible enhancement and thickening of the cisternal segment of the oculomotor nerve on contrast-enhanced MR images. *AJNR Am J Neuroradiol* 1998;19:1887–91, copyright © American Society of Neuroradiology (www.ajnr.org)

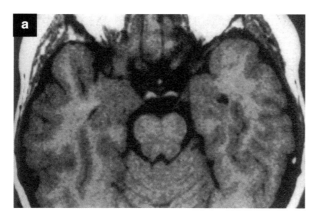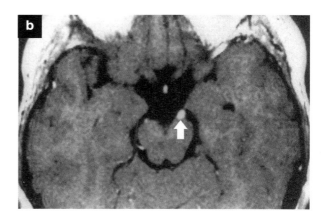

Figure 8.33 Twelve-year-old boy with two prior episodes of ophthalmoplegic migraine. (a) and (b), axial T1-weighted MR images before (a) and after (b) contrast administration show enhancement of the oculomotor nerve (arrow in panel b) and thickening of its root entry zone. Follow-up studies showed virtually complete resolution of the enhancement. Reproduced with permission from Mark AS, Casselman J, Brown D, *et al.* Ophthalmoplegic migraine: Reversible enhancement and thickening of the cisternal segment of the oculomotor nerve on contrast-enhanced MR images. *AJNR Am J Neuroradiol* 1998;19:1887–91, copyright © American Society of Neuroradiology (www.ajnr.org)

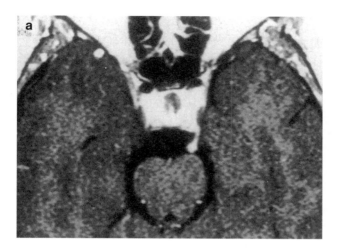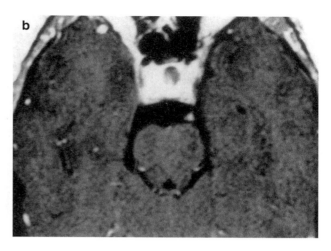

Figure 8.34 Twenty-three-year-old woman with one prior episode of ophthalmoplegic migraine. (a) axial T1-weighted contrast-enhanced MR image shows enhancement of the oculomotor nerve and thickening of its root entry zone; (b) follow-up study shows virtually complete resolution of the enhancement. Reproduced with permission from Mark AS, Casselman J, Brown D, *et al.* Ophthalmoplegic migraine: Reversible enhancement and thickening of the cisternal segment of the oculomotor nerve on contrast-enhanced MR images. *AJNR Am J Neuroradiol* 1998;19:1887–91, copyright © American Society of Neuroradiology (www.ajnr.org)

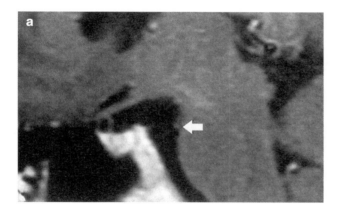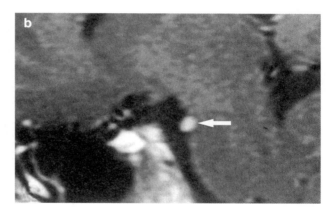

Figure 8.35 Eight-year-old girl with one prior episode of spontaneously resolving oculomotor nerve palsy. (a) and (b), sagittal T1-weighted MR image before (a) and after (b) contrast administration show focal thickening and enhancement of the root exit zone (see arrows). The symptoms resolved spontaneously within 6 weeks. Reproduced with permission from Mark AS, Casselman J, Brown D, *et al.* Ophthalmoplegic migraine: Reversible enhancement and thickening of the cisternal segment of the oculomotor nerve on contrast-enhanced MR images. *AJNR Am J Neuroradiol* 1998;19:1887–91, copyright © American Society of Neuroradiology (www.ajnr.org)

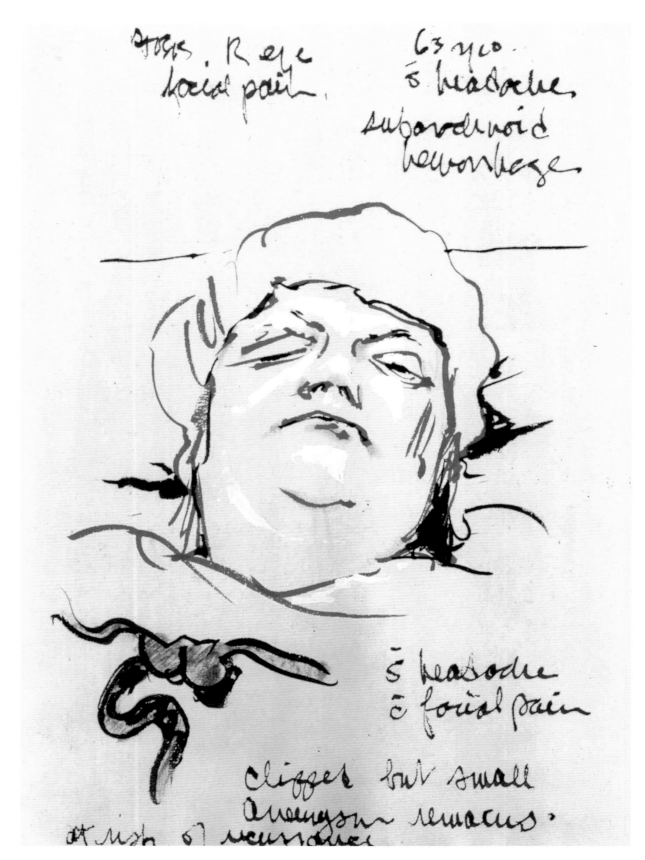

Figure 8.36 Sixty-three-year-old female presents with right eye pain and ptosis. Patient diagnosed with subarachnoid hemorrhage and an aneurysm was discovered and clipped. Reproduced with kind permission of Gary Carpenter

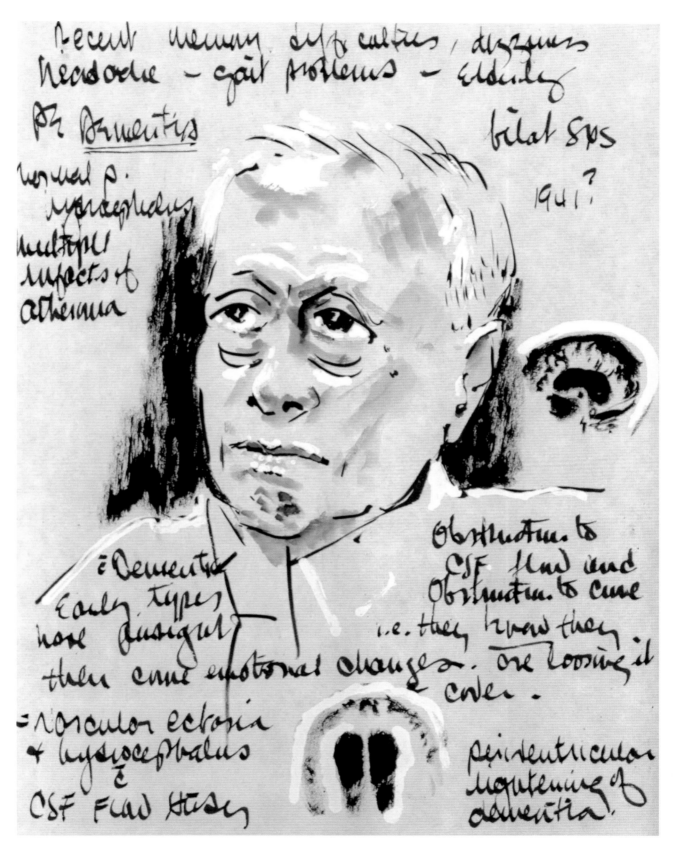

Figure 8.37 Elderly patient presents with complaint of recent memory difficulties, dizziness, headache and gait disturbances. Patient found to have obstruction of cerebrospinal fluid flow with large ventricles and periventricular leucomalacia. Reproduced with kind permission of Gary Carpenter

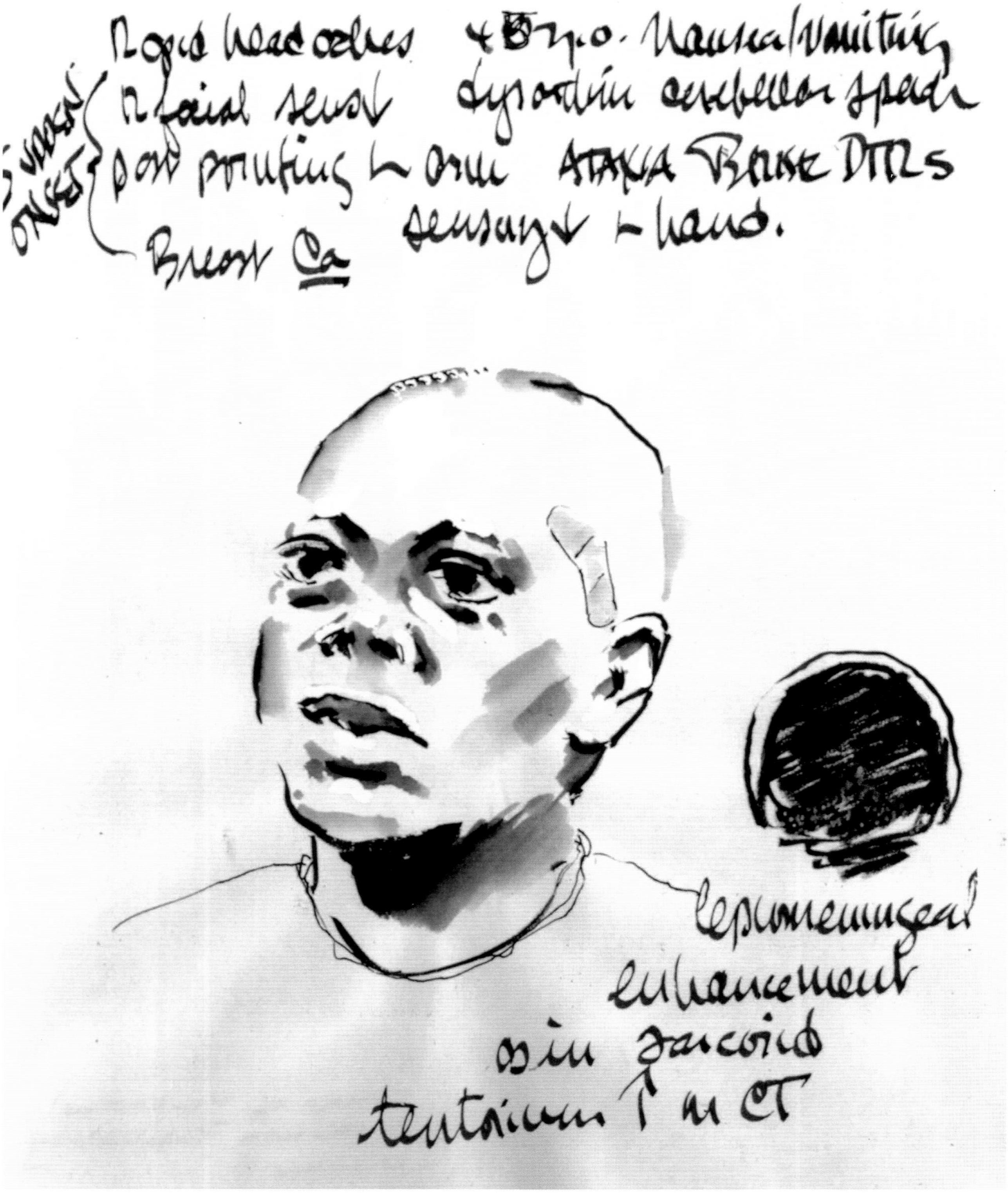

Figure 8.38 Forty-year-old female presents with sudden-onset, right-sided headache with nausea and vomiting, decreased right facial sensation, dysarthria, partial pointing of right arm, ataxia, increased deep tendon reflexes and sensory loss in left hand. Patient had history of breast cancer and CT showed leptomeningeal enhancement in tentorium consistent with carcinomatous meningitis. Reproduced with kind permission of Gary Carpenter

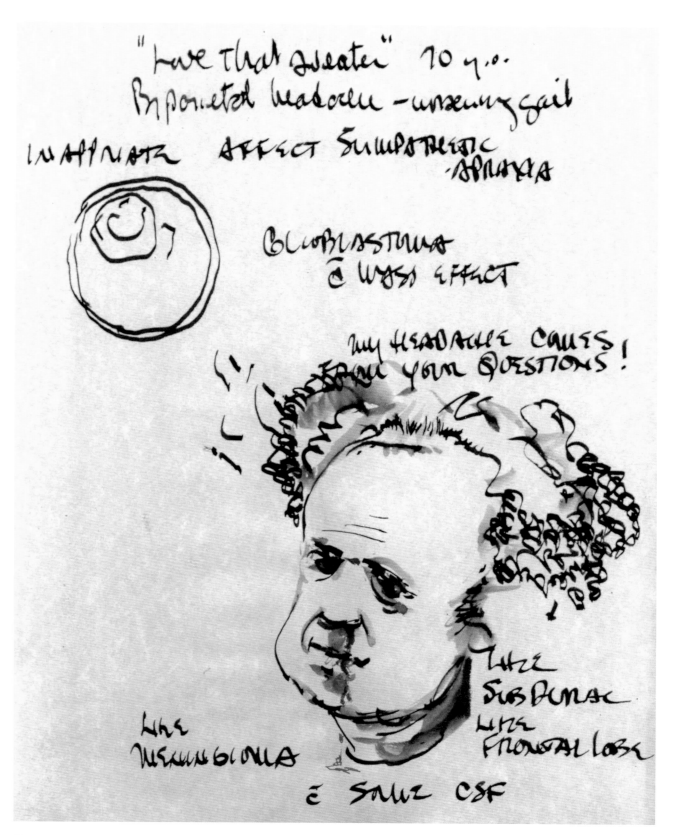

Figure 8.39 Seventy-year-old male presents with bilateral parietal headache and unsteady gait. Patient also has inappropriate affect and apraxia. Patient is found to have right frontal lobe glioblastoma with mass effect and developed a cerebrospinal fluid leak postoperatively. Reproduced with kind permission of Gary Carpenter

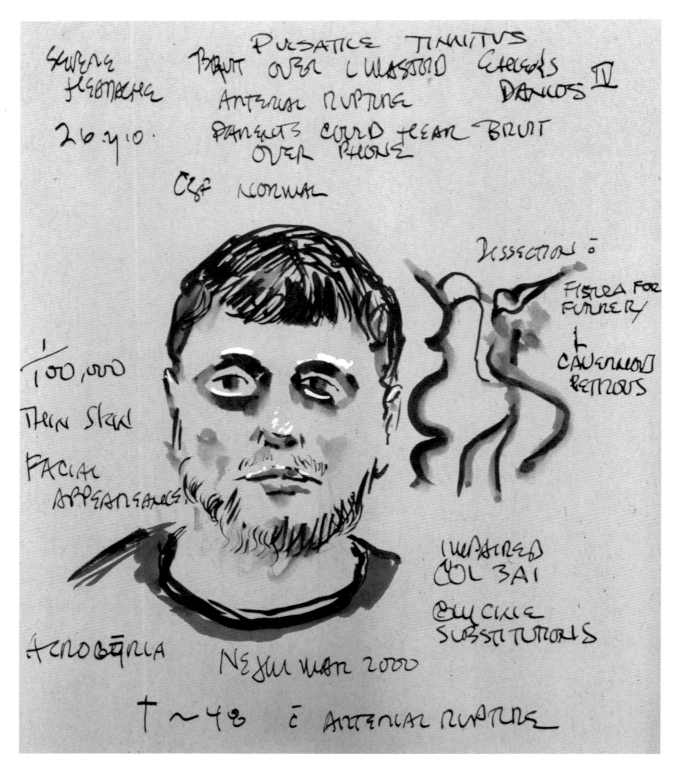

Figure 8.40 Twenty-six-year-old male presents with severe headache and pulsatile tinnitus. Bruits were auscultated over left carotid artery. Bruit was loud enough at times to be heard over the telephone. Cerebrospinal fluid exam was negative. Patient found to have carotid dissection anterior rupture and fistula with left cavernous sinus. Patient is thin with acrogyria. Reproduced with kind permission of Gary Carpenter

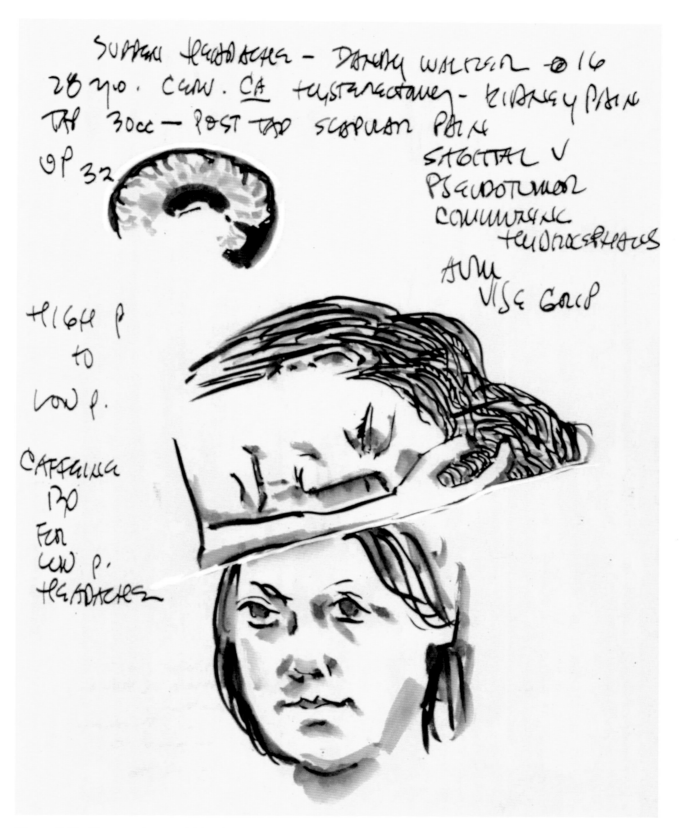

Figure 8.41 Twenty-eight-year-old female with a history of Dandy–Walker syndrome diagnosed at age 16 presents with sudden onset headache. Opening pressure of lumbar puncture was 32 cm H$_2$O. After lumbar puncture patient developed scapula pain and headache when in upright position. Patient had high pressure to low pressure headache after the lumbar puncture and was treated with caffeine. Reproduced with kind permission of Gary Carpenter

Index